DESTINED FOR GREATNESS

Copyright Notice

DESTINED FOR GREATNESS

Copyright © 2017 Shantay Carter, All rights reserved, including the right to reproduce this book or portion thereof in any form whatsoever.

This book is designed to provide accurate and authoritative information with regard to the subject matter covered. It is sold with the understanding that there is not a professional consulting engagement. If legal or other expert advice or assistance is required please seek a licensed professional in your area.

For information on bulk orders or to have Shantay Carter speak at your event, contact : woiinc2011@gmail.com

Table of Contents:

Shantay Carter BSN, RN ....
    Destined For Greatness 1

Professor Renalda T. Carter MSN, RN ....
    Business, Healthcare, Law And Nursing 18

Venus Ricks, RN ....
    From RN to CEO: CHANGING LANES 38

Michelle G. Rhodes MHS, RN ....
    THE NURSE ENTREPRENEUR COLLECTIVE 59

Jeteia L. Benson RN, MSN, FNP-C ....
    WHEN NURSING ISN'T ENOUGH................................78

BRITTANY WINESTOCK APRN, FNP-BC ....
    TRUSTING MY JOURNEY: Inspirational Stories of Nurse Entrepreneurs 96

Melanie McCrary-Fuller BSN, RN ....
    FROM SCRUBS TO PUMPS...114

Shawanna Guillory, FNP-BC ....
   BEAUTY, BRAINS, AND BUSINESS 125

Lakesha Reed-Curtis MSN, RN ....
   ALWAYS ON DUTY 142

Tiffany Jackson, LPN ....
   THE JOURNEY: NURSING AND BEYOND 157

References 171

DEDICATION

I would like to dedicate this book to all the women who stepped out on faith, followed their dreams, and pursued their passions.

"I've learned that people will forget what you said, people will forget what you did, but people will never forget how you made them feel. If you don't like something, change it. If you can't change it, change your attitude. There is no greater agony than bearing an untold story inside you."

-Dr. Maya Angelou

First and foremost, I would like to thank God for his continuous favor and blessings in my life. I am very thankful because I come from a family with strong spiritual values. Faith and work played a major part in my family's decision making and it plays a major part in mine today.

I come from a family of Jamaican descent. In the 1970's, there were not a lot of opportunities in my family's native country of Jamaica; however, my grandmother was determined to leave a legacy that would last for generations. Her goal was to give her children and grandchildren opportunities she did not have as a child. As a result, my grandmother stepped out on faith by leaving Jamaica to come and pursue the American Dream. When she came to the United States, she worked three and four jobs to make ends meet as a single mother so she could take care of her four kids. My grandmother was determined, dedicated, and disciplined; and she instilled those same work ethics in me. One of the reasons I follow my passions and desires is because my grandmother was my example and role model. She drilled in me the importance of getting my education and working hard. I would like to thank my grandmother for her hard work and the sacrifices she made for her family. More importantly, I would like to thank my grandmother for helping me to become the woman that I am today.

I would also like to thank my parents. My parents always believed in me and they supported my dreams. At an early age, my mom, Marcia Smith Hart, taught me that if you are in a position where you can help others, especially those who are less fortunate, then you should. My mom taught me the act of being selfless by her giving heart, endless love, and warm hugs. I am very grateful to have been blessed with such a loving and supportive mother.

My dad, Patrick Carter, taught me to never settle for less and to never give up because being a failure was not an option for me. He taught me to be tenacious when I needed to be and to always stay focused on my goals.

I would also like to thank my extended family for believing in me and supporting me since the beginning of my life. I truly appreciate each and every one of them. I would especially like to thank the ones who helped me to pay for Women of Integrity's 501C 3; to them, I am forever grateful.

I want to thank my Girls, better known as my support system. Thanks for supporting me from day one. To my Bestie Ayanna, thank you for helping me come up with the name Women of Integrity. The name stuck, and look how far we've come 7 years later. Thanks for putting up with my late-night calls to you guys about my frustration and fears of starting my own business. Most importantly, thanks for always reassuring me that I got this. I love all of you ladies.

Last but not least, I want to thank my business mentor Racquel. She guided me in the early stages of creating Women of Integrity Inc. Racquel was a successful business owner herself, but she took the time out of her busy schedule to mentor me and guide me into the right direction.

Destined For Greatness

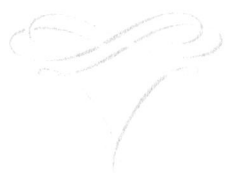

BY
Shantay Carter BSN, RN

INTRODUCTION

My name is Shantay Yolanda Carter, the only child born to Marcia Smith and Patrick Carter. I am a Registered Nurse and the Founder of Women Of Integrity Inc. I am a member of Alpha Kappa Alpha Sorority, Incorporated and a member of Black Nurses Rock, Inc. My family is from Jamaica, West Indies; my grandmother came to the United States with her four children to make a better way of life for them all. Growing up, I always admired my grandmother. She was this beautiful, strong, and hard working woman. She was the first person I knew to work in healthcare. I always loved seeing her in her crisp white uniform going to work. She always expressed such a great sense of pride when it came to her work. She enjoyed helping others and was always willing to do so if she could. The importance of getting an education, doing well in school, and having manners was always stressed in my household. Looking back now, I can say that my grandmother undoubtedly inspired me. Growing up I was blessed to have an amazing support system, which was my family. I grew up in a house filled with strong and beautiful women who taught me to be independent, strong, resilient, kind, educated, and to always carry myself like a lady.

My journey to becoming the woman and nurse that I am today wasn't an easy one. I made a lot of mistakes growing up.

When I was younger, I went through a rebellious teenager phase. During that phase, I got into a lot of trouble in school. I would have to go to in-school suspension for days at a time. After a while, it started to get boring and began to wear on me. At that point I realized that I had to do better if I ever wanted to graduate and make something of myself. Being considered the rebel or the disobedient kid was not the title that I wanted to hold. I got my act together by the time I started high school. I graduated with honors and was in the top of my class. At first I wanted to become a Neurosurgeon, because I wanted to help find a cure for the type of brain cancer from which my Grandmother (my dad's mom) died. In high school, math was not my strong suit. After speaking with my HS Guidance Counselor, he advised me to go into nursing instead. Deciding to become a Registered Nurse was one the best decisions I ever made.

I got accepted into the Nursing program at Binghamton University after graduating high school. My college years was one of the best times of my life. During those four years of college, I started to figure out who I was and what kind of woman I wanted to be. In nursing school, I learned that there is no such thing as an excuse; to make it in life, you had to work very hard. As a woman of color, I had to work twice as hard. It also meant that there would be some sacrifices that I would have to make. While in nursing school, I had to deal with instructors who didn't believe in me and told me I would never become a Nurse. Once they let me know that they doubted me, it only made me work harder to prove my worth and become a Nurse. I graduated on time with my BSN in Nursing. Nursing school taught me discipline, which also helped me in other aspects of my life. I went to one of the top Nursing schools in the country, which made sure I was well prepared for my nursing career. My takeaways from Nursing school are the following: everything you do and don't do affects your patient; and never apologize for being thorough or for advocating for your patient.

While attending Binghamton, I also worked as a Resident Assistant. Working as a Resident Assistant was truly a rewarding experience because it taught me how to work with other people from different races and cultures. The RA position helped to develop my leadership and people skills, which would help me in nursing and later prepare me for my current role as Founder of Women Of Integrity Inc. As an RA, I also learned how to plan programs and workshops for the students. I had to work with my other fellow RA's to make sure the residence hall ran smoothly and that we were keeping the students informed and safe. I currently work at one the top hospitals on Long Island. Just think, I was told I would never become a Nurse. My haters served as my motivators. I have been a Registered Nurse for seventeen years now, and I love it . I love my profession and I love helping people.

Nursing has given me the opportunity to grow and help identify the areas of need in our communities. Becoming a Registered Professional Nurse also helped with disciplining my work practices. I always strive to do what is right and best for my patient as opposed to what is easy and fast. I am extremely thorough and a slight perfectionist when it comes to my work as Nurse and my work in the community. Working with different populations taught me that even if we look different on the outside, we as women all go through similar things. Women are the backbones of our families and communities; women are the key. So, if you empower and educate our women, it will lead to better families and better communities. This is just one of the many reasons I wanted to start my own business, so that I could be of service to other women. When I was growing up, I saw many of my peers get pregnant at an early age or drop out of high school. Then later in life, I saw them trying to go back to school to get their education or working low paying jobs and struggling. That always made me wonder, like what could've been done differently in their lives. In this day and time and even when I was growing up, there were so many potential obstacles that could get in the way of a young girl's life. Whether it was boy trouble, sex, abuse, drugs, alcohol, or a troubled childhood. If you didn't have a strong, affirmative support system, you would end up another Black Girl lost. I have always wanted to work with and help those women that may be less fortunate. Being a Nurse also means it is in my nature to want to help people. As a woman it is in my nature to be a nurturer.

In 2010, I had gone through a very bad breakup. I was with this person for over five years. Towards the end, the relationship became very toxic; it had taken a toll on me emotionally and spiritually. After the breakup, I was at a low point in my life. I had lost all my self-worth; heck, I didn't feel as if I was worthy of anything or anyone. During that dark time, I was consumed with a lot of anger, hurt, and feelings of betrayal. This negative energy began to affect my relationships at work and with my family and friends. People did not want to be around me. I started staying to myself a lot and stayed locked in my room. It's hard to give your all to someone just to get nothing back in return, and be made to feel that you were never good enough or just enough. Looking back now, I was probably depressed then and didn't know it. Sometimes mental abuse can be worse than any of the other forms of abuse. Once you break a person mentally, it's hard to come back from that. I knew I had to change my life around, stop playing the victim role, take responsibility for my role in certain things, be honest with myself, and channel that negative energy into something positive. I had to turn my pain into power. I was blessed and fortunate to have real friends and family that were truly supportive and helped me get through that time in my life.

As a means of channeling that negative energy into something positive, I started to think of all the things that I wanted to do in my life but had never got the chance. One thing I remembered that I always wanted to do was to start an organization that would help young girls and women. One night in my basement, I came up with the idea to finally start my women's organization. I always knew that I wanted to give back to my community and work with young girls. I wanted to create a group that would be comprised of like-minded, positive women from all different backgrounds. I decided to create Women Of Integrity Inc. (WOI) was created to give back to my community and channel that negative energy into something positive. I picked the name Women Of Integrity Inc., because I felt that it was a powerful name and when people heard it, they would want to know what we're about. My best friend Ayanna helped me come up with the name, and we voted on it as a group and that name won. I want WOI to be the support system for the lost and often misguided girls. I am a firm believer that what you put out in life, you get back; therefore, if you put out positivity, you will get back positivity.

> "The positive thinker sees the invisible, feels the intangible, and achieves the impossible."
>
> -Winston Churchill

I TURNED MY PAIN INTO MY POWER, WHICH LED ME TO MY PURPOSE

Becoming a Nurse Entrepreneur was not something that I planned. It happened out of the need for me to change my life. Creating Women Of Integrity Inc. saved my life. It has helped me to become a better woman, friend, daughter, sister, and Nurse. Women Of Integrity Inc. helped heal me mentally. It made me realize my own self-worth and understand that you should never allow someone else to validate you; only you can validate yourself.

On November 30th, 2010, I Founded Women Of Integrity Inc., a nonprofit organization geared towards empowering and educating women of all ages and ethnicities. We started out as a group on Facebook. I invited all my family and friends to be a part of the group. Based on everyone's feedback, we decided that we wanted to mentor young girls and do service projects which would allow us to give back to our community. As time went on, we grew from a Facebook group to an actual functioning organization.

In the beginning, the process was tough. It was tough getting support from the community. It was hard to even get my organization incorporated. It took me three tries before I got it right. They sent back my paperwork three times and I was starting to feel discouraged. I reached out to my cousin who had a business at the time and another cousin who had who worked with government. They helped revise my application for my incorporation papers. As they say, the third time's the charm! We became incorporated on September 23rd, 2011. This was definitely a happy moment for the organization and me.

OUR MISSION STATEMENT

Women Of Integrity Inc.- is an organization of diverse women spanning different educational, racial, and socio-economic backgrounds. Our aim is to support and empower girls, adolescents, and women by fostering the confidence and nurturing the skills necessary to accomplish their goals, dreams, and aspirations of the future.

We extend our support through: Volunteer service, Professional mentoring programs, and community outreach events.

I learned along the way to never be afraid to ask for help. For my first prom dress drive, we only collected ten dresses. I literally cried to my mom like no one donated to us at all. How are we going to help the girls in need? I remember my mom saying, "You just have to give it time. People don't know who you are right now, so don't get discouraged." From that experience, I learned that I had to go out there and network and inform the community about who we were and what we represented. The lack of dresses donated our first year gave me the idea to later create our Prom Makeover Project.

For the last seven years, I have been grinding and putting in the work required to help make my business successful and grow. The grind never stops and I am constantly working on my business. WOI has hosted many different programs for the community. Our signature events are our annual prom dress drive, prom dress giveaway, and annual prom makeover project. We have given away hundreds of free prom dresses over the years, helping to make prom dreams come true for underserved girls. With our prom makeover project, we make over a high school senior for her prom. In the prom makeover package, we provide the hair, makeup, dress, shoes, accessories, and a professional photographer. We are essentially that girl's glam squad for the day. The look on the young lady's face, as we pamper her on her prom day is priceless. It is such a rewarding feeling that we are able to help a young lady go to prom. Every young girl deserves to go to their prom, especially if they have worked hard in school. Going to prom, is one of those rites of passage moments that every girl should experience despite whether or not they can financially afford it. This is where our annual free prom dress giveaway and prom makeover project come into play.

We have hosted etiquette, financial education, and healthy living workshops. My role as a Nurse is to educate my community as well. I try to incorporate the importance of healthy living through our health workshops. I think it is important to teach our young women about etiquette and carrying themselves like a lady. Financial education is an important topic for our community to learn.

My favorite aspect of the organization is the mentoring portion. This is where we get to work with a local high school's after-school mentoring program. The girls range from 9th-12th grade. We meet on a weekly basis with the girls. We speak to the girls on an array of different topics. We always stress to them the importance of education, self-worth, and self-love. We let them know that once you have your education, no one can take that from you; and when you have your education, you become empowered; when you're empowered, you can change the world. I have kept in contact with many of my mentees over the years. They know that they can still call me whenever they need to talk. My door is always open to them.

For the last two years, we have hosted our annual Women in Business Networking Brunch with the local Chamber of Commerce. We wanted to add a new program and the Women in Business networking Brunch allowed us to tap into that market of women who are looking to start a business or grow their existing business. At this event we have an amazing lineup of panelist, to answer every and all things business. The women also get to network with other like-minded women. At the end of the event they are leaving empowered and educated, which is the goal of our events and the organization.

In 2015, we received our 501C 3 status, which was such a big accomplishment. It took us five years to receive our tax-exempt status., but we never lost faith or gave up on the process. Achieving our tax-exempt status allowed doors that may have been closed before to now open. It allows us a seat at the table in certain arenas. It also makes the community look at you more seriously. Everyone's process and journey will be different. You must respect and trust your process. This year we will celebrate our seven-year anniversary. We have come such a long way. I had to grind to gain visibility for my organization. Networking is very important, but networking with the right people is priceless. Collaborating with other people and organizations can be helpful as well to gain visibility and get your name out there. Just remember when collaborating with other people, you want to make sure their agenda is aligned with your mission and purpose. In the beginning, we had no community support; but now seven years later, the support from the community is amazing and such a rewarding feeling. Women Of Integrity Inc. has grown into a successful organization. Our work in the community speaks for itself.

What has been most rewarding since starting WOI, is the impact that we have made in our community and the impact we have had on the girls lives that we have come in contact with. The priceless faces when they find the right prom dress or when they win the prom makeover project contest. When I look back at our humble beginnings and see how far we have come and all that we have achieved, has been nothing but a blessing. You have to be a blessing in order to receive a blessing.

There were many challenges that I have had to face during my journey of creating WOI. Then there are those challenges that you have to face on a day-to-day basis. I have had other organizations try to come after WOI , saying that we were using their name. Our names were similar , but the not the same. That other organization went as far as writing on our Facebook wall, being disrespectful and trying to tell us to take down our page. When that incident happened , I decided to hire an attorney to represent WOI. My attorney sent out a cease and desist letter to the organization. I have not heard from them again. I strongly encourage everyone to get a lawyer, if you can. Remember , you have to always protect your brand and your business. Two of my worst experiences since starting WOI was, having one man make inappropriate sexual advances, and another man talking down to me, and trying to belittle me at a business meeting. The first incident, involved a man I looked up to and who had also opened doors for WOI. I went to have a meeting with him and next thing I know he was groping himself in front of me and telling me he would give me money , in essence in return for sexual favors. I was so shocked, I got up and walked out of there in disbelief . He tried to apologize, but I would not accept it and cut all ties and affiliations with him. I was so disgusted that a man I once trusted and respected would try to take advantage of me. That experience taught me that I have to set boundaries, and make it very clear to people what I will and won't allow.

The second incident was where I was at a business meeting to discuss a possible interview with a radio show. The man who set up the meeting began to discuss the details of the interview. As he began to discuss the fees, I interrupted him and reminded him that he never once mentioned any fees. After I said that, the man began to raise his voice at me , all the while speaking in a condescending tone. I was the only female in the room. I could tell by their body language, that the other men in the room started to become uncomfortable with the way the man was speaking to me. At that point , I kindly got up and let him know that he will not speak to me in that manner and walked out. After that I learned, that I had to start commanding respect from my male counterparts, and start learning to ask the right questions before agreeing to anything.

The most challenging thing since starting WOI, was to actually start it. For years , I put the idea on the back burner out of fear. I was afraid that I could not pull it off. Once I finally faced that fear and stepped out on faith, everything else fell into place. My day-to-day struggles deal with the sacrifices that I have to make in order to grow my business. One of biggest struggles now is trying to balance work life, family, friends, personal, and business. My family and friends say that I am always so busy, and that I have no time for them. I am also single . I feel like certain things had to be put off, so that I could focus on WOI. The grind and the hustle is real, and if you don't put in that work, you will not see results. I say all this to say that, the good that comes out of the work that you do, will always outweigh the bad. Every obstacle that you face, or every sacrifice that you have to make , will just make you journey even better when you reach your goal. I have learned now most recently that it's ok to stop and smell the roses along your journey and just live in that moment.

My Legacy, what would I want that to be? I have always said from the beginning, " If I am able to just help one girl, then I have done my job". I would want people to remember Women Of Integrity Inc., and myself for the work that we did in our community. My vision for the organization, is to eventually become a nationally recognized organization with chapters in other states. As well as becoming a premier community resource and support system for the women and young women in my community.

To my fellow Nurses who want to start to a business, remember starting a business is never easy. In the beginning, I had the support of my family and friends; but as time went on, I lost the support of some of those same people. One of the biggest things I had to learn was that I can't take things personal. My vision and my dream is not going to necessarily be everyone else's dream. Everybody is not meant to be a part of my journey. Once I learned that, I wasn't afraid anymore to grow and understand that I may lose people along the way. It made me stronger. It taught me that sometimes you must go outside your comfort zone. It also taught me to never become too dependent on one person or thing. If you know in your heart that you want to start a business, then go for it. Do your research, figure out your purpose or what you are passionate about , and then let your creative juices flow. If you never try, you will never know, and not knowing is worse than failing.

All these experiences in my life and Nursing have helped mold me into the businesswoman that I am today. I am a stronger woman today than I was seven years ago, because of WOI. I am a woman that knows who she is and where she is going. I have learned to love myself and know my worth. If you don't love yourself or know your worth, you can't expect anyone else to know. I have found my purpose and I am walking in it. My purpose is to help other women, especially young women. Once you find your purpose, your vision for your business will become clear. You just have to remain focused, believe in yourself, and never let anyone dull your shine. These are ten key points I have learned along the way and would like to share:

MY 10 KEY TAKEAWAY POINTS

Lesson 1: Knowledge is key and knowledge is power.

Lesson 2: In life you will always have the naysayers and haters, but how you react to them is what makes all the difference.

Lesson 3: You must be willing to put in the work that is required for you to succeed. Also, self-promotion is one of the best forms of promotion.

Lesson 4: Always believe in yourself and your dream because if you don't believe in your dream, how can you expect anyone else to believe in it.

Lesson 5: Your network determines your net worth. Don't be afraid to network and make new business connections.

Lesson 6: Never give up because failure is not an option. Every setback is a setup for a comeback.

Lesson 7: Research your industry. Make sure there is a need for your business. Research your competition, if there is any. No sense in reinventing wheel. Just figure out what can you do to make your business stand out.

Lesson 8: Always have an attitude of gratitude. Be Humble, and don't be afraid to ask for help.

Lesson 9: Find your purpose and walk in it. Figure out what you are passionate about or what makes you happy and do that.

Lesson 10: Whatever your business is, if your heart is not in it, you will not win. It is your passion/purpose, and faith that will keep you going.

My final tip is: surround yourself with positive people. Find your dream team. In order to grow your business, you will need a team. Picking the right people to be a part of your team can either make or break your business.

I want to thank all the people that believed in me and supported me from day one until now. I truly appreciate each and every one of you. I pray that I will be able to continue to serve my community for years to come. I am glad that I was given this opportunity to share my experiences, because my goal is to have others be able to learn from my journey.

Shantay Carter

"Service to others is the rent you pay for your room here on earth"

-Muhammad Ali

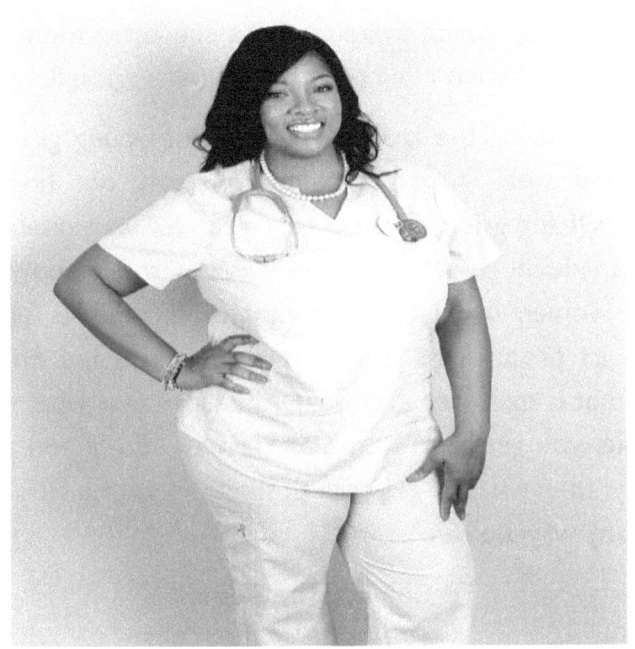

About the Author

When it comes to Shantay Carter, helping others is more than just a job—it's her passion and her purpose. From her daily work as a dedicated nurse to her ambitions as founder of Women Of Integrity Inc., the New York area native has an extensive history of letting her caring nature guide her path.

Influenced strongly by the superwoman role models in her family, Shantay decided to dive head first into the nursing field. After spending years selflessly volunteering as a candy striper while in high school, she headed to Binghamton University where she received a Bachelor of Science degree in Nursing. In 2000, she began working at Binghamton General Hospital as a registered nurse and in 2002, Shantay continued her career at North Shore-LIJ Health System where she currently works as an Orthopedic/Bariatric nurse on a medical/surgical floor.

After noticing the lack of guidance for young girls in the Long Island area, Shantay decided to create her non-profit, Women Of Integrity Inc. The four-year-old organization has already made huge strides in its mission to "empower and educate women of all ages and ethnicities" and its signature event is its prom dress drive, dress giveaway, and makeover project that is executed each year. "I believe that what you put out in life, you get back," explains Shantay. "So, if you put out positivity, then you will get back positivity— it's our job to give back in any way we can."

To Contact The Author:

www.womenofintegrityinc.org

IG: @WOIINC & S.Carterrn

FB: facebook.com/WOIINC

Business, Healthcare, Law AND Nursing

BY
Professor Renalda T. Carter MSN, RN

FINDING MY PURPOSE

I can honestly say my career in the healthcare field has resulted in true purpose driven success! I always knew I was going to own my own business however, I did not know what that business was going to be. I did know working for other people was not going to allow me to have the control over my life I would need to be truly happy. I am now the Founder and Senior Consultant at RTC Legal Nurse Consulting, LLC. I am also the Professor of Healthcare Law and Ethics at Harris-Stowe State University Anheuser-Bush School of Business. My students always want to know what it was like when I was in school and how I was able to become a successful educator. When I tell them the story the students are quiet as mice. They love to hear the lessons and tips I have learned along the way and how I used my nursing skills to build a business in healthcare law. The students are the ones that asked me to write this book. I hope my journey will benefit anyone interested in owning their own business.

As a young girl, I dreamed of operating a huge company and living in a large mansion with a pool, tennis court, and a spa. I had visions of driving a Lamborghini, wearing a fierce business suit, carrying my briefcase and looking like a real Boss. I had planned to build a business that would support my entire family for generations to come. Well, it turns out, that was going to be easier said than done.

While my friends were off enjoying their teenage years, I spent my days planning how to make becoming a business owner a reality. One particular day, I was in the kitchen listening to the radio and there was an advertisement about how to become successful. The advertisement said, all I had to do was go to Professional Business School (PBS). That sounded like a great plan to me as a teenager and just like that, it was decided. I would graduate from high school, go to Professional Business School (PBS) and then start my own company.

My senior year in high school, I met my husband. I was eighteen years old. We went out on double dates with our friends, went to prom together and before I knew it, we were married and parents. In my defense, prior to the wedding, I did graduate from high school and completed Professional Business School as planned. I learned computer skills that were in high demand at that time but I did not learn how to operate my own business. I received a certificate to work as a Computer Operator.

My husband decided to leave college early and we both signed up to work for a temporary agency. The agency put me to work full-time as a computer operator and my husband worked in construction. It looked like we were going to live happily ever after. In my mind, I knew it would only be a matter of time before we owned our own family business.

The pay at the agency was appreciated but the daycare expenses exceeded my pay and we decided I would stay home with our son until he was old enough to go to school. All of my high school friends had gone off to college and although I loved my family, being at home all day became a real challenge. I also started to notice subtle changes in my husband's behavior. He began to act and move in a different way. We were unable to keep up with the bills on his salary alone, so we had to move in with his mom. I felt bad living with his mom and not being able to contribute to the household expenses so I decided to have a family member keep our child for free and signed up to work for the agency again. They had jobs posted for a secretary and a telemarketer. I did both.

I met a lot of people while working for agency but one girl stood out. Her name was Patricia Hudson. Patricia told me she was tired of being broke, living from paycheck to paycheck and she was going to apply to work at a nursing home. Patricia's mom had worked in the field for years and now Patricia was going to become a Certified Nurse Assistant (CNA) as well. Patricia went on to say, the nursing home would pay employees just to learn to become a Certified Nurse Assistant (CNA). That's when my journey to becoming a Nurse Entrepreneur started.

NURSING

I had never seen the inside of a nursing home before and the things I saw during the training were truly a culture shock. I wasn't sure if this job was going to work out for me. Patricia continued to encourage me and we attended the classes faithfully. She made the classes fun and we laughed through the hard times. After completing the CNA training, we both passed the written exam and practicum required. The CNA course prepared us for entry-level employment in the nursing home. There was a skilled nursing unit, a residential unit, and an

Alzheimer's unit at the nursing home. I was assigned to work on all of the units.

Some of my duties included bathing residents, making beds, taking vital signs, providing personal care, safe patient lifting, assistance with elimination, performing range of motion and much, much, more. A lot of the elderly residents had Alzheimer's disease. It felt good for me to be able to help people in this way however, I am not the one to settle for the ordinary. No, that is not in my nature. I was always exploring ways to enhance my skills and increase my earning potential to help others on a larger scale.

Within six months of working as a CNA, I decided to enroll in an evening class to become a Certified Medication Technician (CMT). I became proficient in the administration of many types of medications and was required to perform this task to assist licensed practical nurses (LPN) and/or a Registered Professional Nurses (RN) in medication therapy. I also learned to transcribe or copy physician orders, observe, report and document medication side effects using approved medical terminology and abbreviations. After two years of working for nursing homes and observing the responsibilities of the nurses, I realized this was my road to acquiring the business that I always dreamed of having. It was time for me to take on additional responsibilities by enrolling in a Licensed Practical Nurse (LPN) training program. I had a new vision. I could clearly see a successful career in the healthcare field.

The admission process for the LPN program was competitive. Successful applicants were selected on the basis of test scores, recommendations, and an interview. Having said that, I passed the admission test without a problem and subsequently attended the Saint Louis Board of Education Practical Nursing Program. I selected this school because, The Missouri State Board of Nursing approved the LPN program, the school's pass rate was over 90%, and the cost was reasonable. During my training as an LPN, all my previous skills as a CNA and CMT were reinforced and I also learned how to perform a head-to-toe assessment, administer injections, administration of medication through a gastrointestinal tube, insertion of a catheter, along with many other clinical skills. This program helped build problem solving and critically thinking skills as well. \ I met several new friends and we had the time of our lives. We all graduated from the LPN program and all passed the NCLEX-PN exam. I was able to become a Charge Nurse, Clinical Supervisor, CNA Instructor, CMT Instructor, Assistant Director of Nursing and later, a Director of Nursing.

RESIDENTIAL CARE FACILITY (RCF) NURSE

In addition to working in nursing homes, I decided to explore other career opportunities. The first position I acquired outside of working in the nursing home was at a Residential Care Facility (RCF). I was confident and prepared to deliver safe, patient-centered care as an entry-level nurse. This position allowed me to focus on residents with various behavioral health disorders. The residents were adults and none of them had Alzheimer's. Getting to know each resident was a pleasure. I was responsible for administering medication and assisting the medical doctor with the therapeutic programs ordered. I was also responsible for monitoring the residents for abnormal behavior, documenting the behavior and contacting the doctor when necessary. I truly enjoyed this position. I learned, working at a RCF requires a gifted and skill worker. The worker must be patient and always ready for the unknown. There are individual treatment plans and the nurse must be aware of each treatment plan. In addition to caring for the residents, I was allowed to function in a supervisory role, acting as a mentor for the Certified Nurse Assistants and Certified Medication Technicians.

My trajectory to success continued when I enrolled at the Saint Louis Florissant Valley Community College to obtain an Associate of Applied Science (AAS) Degree in Nursing. The AAS program prepares students to sit for the National Council Licensure Examination (NCLEX-RN). Passing this exam grants an individual the permission to practice nursing in the state where he or she satisfied the requirements. The National Council of State Boards of Nursing, Inc. (NCSBN) owns and develops the NCLEX-RN examination to ensure and determine if it is safe for the individual to begin practice as a registered nurse. Licensed Practical Nurses from all over came here to become Registered Nurses. I became friends with a lady named, Dana France. Dana was an LPN at the Veterans Administration Hospital. She had been and LPN for ten years and was proficient at most of the skills we were still trying to achieve. We all looked up to Dana and she helped myself and the other LPN's improve our clinical skills. Dana was truly a life safer. Thanks to Dana, I was able to administer intravenous medication, g-tube medication, and pass my class exams. If it had not been for Dana France and the other ladies I met, school would have been extremely difficult. Instead, the classes were fun and exciting. It was easy to connect class information or didactic material to the clinical practicum. Last year, I ran into Dana France at one of the nursing homes I teach my LPN students at. Dana is also teaching healthcare students now. All her students love her too.

OCCUPATIONAL HEALTH NURSE

After graduating from the RN program, I passed the NCLEX-RN and received my AAS degree in nursing. I was finally ready to work as a Registered Professional Nurse (RN). Becoming a Registered Nurse was a huge accomplishment for me. I was young and ready to conquer the world. I decided to leave the nursing homes because I was offered the opportunity to work as an Occupational Health Nurse for a large government plant. Most of my duties required performing pre-employment urine drug screens, hearing/vision test, immunizations, employee illness/injury documentation, return to work forms, research, and planning health and wellness events. Now I was creating wellness workshops for adults and I loved every minute of it. However, the main function of the Occupational Health Nurse is to assess and treat employee illnesses/injuries. This job allowed me to improve my nursing documentation skills and study each illness or injury on a case-by case basis. I was trained for 2 weeks however, the first time I was left alone in the office to care for patients with no other nurses or a doctor, I was scared to death! I knew if an employee became injured, it was up to me to make the right call. I was on my own.

I treated at least 50 patients a day. Each day, employees would come to the clinic and sit at my desk to tell me about an injury or illness that had occurred. My job was to document the subjective complaints, make a nursing assessment, treat the problem and evaluate the situation. I was able to really focus on the different disease processes and how they truly present-the clinical picture became real.

I never knew what was going to come through that door. One patient might need some medication for a headache another may need a simple blood pressure check. I also knew there was always the possibility things could go really wrong at any given time. Therefore, I kept my trusty nursing books and the internet at my fingertips to assist me with any minor concerns but if the concerns were major, I would contact the company medical doctor or the clinic Administrator. After a while, I felt comfortable with my assessment skills and no longer needed the internet or my nursing books. I was able to assess the situation, treat the problem and document the outcome without skipping a beat. I also continued to work for the agency, which allowed me to work at several other large companies and experience a wide variety of workers' compensation cases.

One day, while listening to soft jazz and reading a book, the one thing I always feared came to be. I received a 911 call over the radio. A worker was unconscious and not breathing and they needed the Nurse! That Nurse was me. I had no time to think. I gathered my emergency bag, the keys to the clinic and headed for the door. There was a worker in a forklift waiting in front of the clinic for me. He was going to take me to the unconscious worker.

As we arrived to the scene, I noticed the worker was blue from head to toe and another worker was giving the worker Cardiopulmonary Resuscitation (CPR). I immediately reached in my bag and pulled out the Automatic External Defibrillator (AED). I checked for a pulse, there was no pulse and the worker was not breathing so I applied the AED as I was trained to do. The AED checked the worker's heart rhythm and sent an electric shock to restore the heart rhythm back to normal. The ambulance and fire truck showed up after this and we continued to provide CPR until the worker was transferred on a stretcher to the hospital. The worker lived! All of the staff that assisted in saving the workers life, including myself was presented with a dinner and the Abbott EMS Lifesaver Award. Occupational health and workers' compensation became my area of expertise! After mastering this field, I decided, it was time to work as a hospital Nurse.

ACUTE CARE AND NURSING

I landed a job at a local hospital and found my home on the telemetry floor. This position was the most intense position I had experienced. During that time, nurses still worked 8-hour shifts. I was assigned to care for five patients per shift on a good day. The work allowed me to really begin to understand the reason I had to learn all the skills I had to endure in the past. As a Registered Nurse, I provided total patient care, assisted doctors with bedside medical procedures, and established relationships with the multidisciplinary hospital team. Nursing is extremely dynamic it is always changing. After a couple of years working as a telemetry Nurse, the hospital started to mandate 12-hour shifts for Nurses. There was a nursing shortage and the 12-hour shifts would help to cover the staffing needs. However, the float pool Nurses continued to work eight hour shifts.

I worked the 12-hour shifts about a year, but decided to float between the hospital floors to gain experience in neurology, cardiac care, intensive care, emergency room care, medical and surgical nursing. Again, with continued hard work, perseverance and one vision -- refusing to forget where I'd come from -- I enrolled at the University of Missouri-Saint Louis where I earned both my undergraduate (BSN) and graduate (MSN) degrees. I was able to work in various management positions at the hospitals, nursing homes, home health care agencies, schools, insurance companies, colleges and universities. My favorite position was working as a Case Manager on each floor at the hospital.

BUSINESS

In 2001, my ex-husband's girlfriend told me she had started a home health care business. She knew that I was a nurse and encouraged me to start one as well. She gave me all the pertinent information and I completed the application process. I attended the mandatory training and took the mandatory test. And just like that, I became an In- Home Healthcare provider for the state of Missouri. My son was 11 years old and a huge help with the home care business. He asked me if I could give his friends a job too. I let his friend pass out the flyers and we knocked on doors of the elderly in our community. My son was hired as the Director of maintenance, his girlfriend worked as my Secretary, and his best friend did odd jobs around the home care business. Several nurses I knew signed up to work as a Home Health Care Nurse. These nurses helped me to secure contracts with local doctors. I must admit, things were going quite well. I did not get the mansion or the Lamborghini I dreamed of but I was able to purchase a really nice home and two vehicles. I enjoyed two vacations per year and was helping the elderly in my community. I was happy and extremely proud to have completed many important goals. Although the business was doing really well, I was not living my purpose. I decided to get a Masters' Degree in Nursing Administration.

HEALTHCARE LAW

I received my Masters' Degree in Nursing Administration and decided with all this knowledge and experience, it was time to activate my master plan. In 2006, I founded RTC Legal Nurse Consulting, LLC (RTCLNC, LLC). I had six months worth of savings and was dedicated to helping others close the widening economic gap that exists between the rich and the working poor. My mission was to produce healthy and well communities. As Administrator and Senior Consultant at RTC Legal Nurse Consulting (RTCLNC, LLC) the first decision I made was to hire a team of advisors. This team included; an attorney, certified public accountant (CPA), grant-writer, marketing consultant, and a host of certified nurse educators. All of the staff were hired on an as-needed basis. My attorney filed the necessary paperwork to get the firm started. He also worked with me to keep all my legal affairs in order. I was required to get business and disability insurance, medical benefits, and apply for a Dun and Bradstreet number. My CPA made sure if there was no money coming in, there was no money going out. She also filed my taxes for the business and put me in contact with someone to set up the business Simplified Employee Pension (SEP). This is a retirement account for business owners.

My marketing consultant was truly a blessing. She created all my business cards, brochures, cards, pens, magnets, and other marketing materials. She also assisted me with helping the students create wellness products in the wellness workshops I teach. My fundraising and contract manager Paul

Onuzuiruke served the firm well with his passion and expertise in philanthropy and fundraising. He respected and always had the interest of the customer first. Paul also had an online magazine I used to write articles for. A creative and divergent thinker, Mr. Onuzuruike always explored, identified and implemented fundraising strategies that resulted in greater financial revenue—using best practices and a wide range of fundraising vehicles. Paul has also written a book called, "The Administrator".

After hiring my team of advisors, the next step I took was to join the American Association of Legal Nurse Consultants (AALNC). Working with this organization was priceless. The primary role of a Legal Nurse Consultant is to evaluate, analyze, and render information and opinions on the delivery of health care and the resulting outcomes. This was no problem for me since I spent several years working in various healthcare related fields. I met several other nurse consultants at the meetings, and I was put in charge of several committees. As a member of the AALNC, I also attended many events where I was able to find job leads.

The first legal case I worked was a toxic tort case. My desk was filled with hundreds of cases that needed to be screened and accompanied by a written report. As a result of working and winning cases, I gained a lot of experience. The experience gave me the confidence to recruit attorneys knowing, I would provide top of the line professional legal nurse consulting services. I recruited four permanent attorney-clients that I still work with today. My attorney-clients will tell you, "Ms. Carter has a sheer dedication and love for perfection-it is her trademark."

Things were fantastic for ten years and then the stock market crashed. I had recently re-financed my house with an adjustable rate mortgage and I had to sell the house before the loan turned upside down. I also noticed there was something different about my neighborhood. The neighborhood looked different and the neighborhood children were acting different. What had happened to my neighborhood? After observing neighborhood children misbehaving and being disrespectful, I became angry. What was going on? I did not know but I was going to find out.

I FOUND MY PURPOSE

I decided to apply for a job as a school nurse. My goal was to teach, motivate, and inspire the students. I wanted to restore my community by empowering the children in my neighborhood. I was hired as needed at a local school as a substitute nurse and a substitute teacher. I made a list of problems the students were having and developed wellness workshops that provided a solution for each problem. The grade school children were extremely receptive to the wellness workshops. I truly enjoyed working with those students because the likelihood for positive change was excellent. The school district thought I did such an excellent job with the children, I was offered a full-time teaching position. They wanted me to teach Health Occupations for the high school students. Accepting a full-time teaching position at a high school required me to go back to school to become a certified educator. I had to juggle online classes, run a business and teach high school students at the same time. I am so glad I did this. Becoming certified made a huge difference in my teaching expertise.

The high school students were not as easy to teach as the elementary school students. I had to remember, never to hold grudges. Although teenagers may look like adults, they are young adults with many different changes going on in their body and in their life. This position allowed me to research the problems high school students were having and create workshops to assist them as well. I was not able to pay bills on the salary of a new high school teacher however, this job turned out to be the job I enjoyed the most. Driven by the desire to empower others, **I had found my purpose!**

I tried to work full-time and operate a business but this was not possible. I had done all I could do at the school and it was time to get back to my business. I was going to grow the business in a different direction. In addition to consulting for attorneys, I was going to provide health and wellness workshops and certified trainers to teach healthcare occupations courses such as ; CNA, CMT, PCT, EKG, LIMA, Insulin Certification and nursing. I realized as a certified educator, business owners needed my services and so did the community. If there is a need, create the service and your business will thrive.

CONCLUSION

In 2013, I negotiated my first professional training contract with a local Healthcare Training Center (HCTC). I simply walked into the office of the owner and gave her my curriculum vitae. The owner was ready to close the training center due to new changes in state policy and did not think she would be able to hire my company to provide any training at her facility. However, I convinced her to hire my business to train her students and promised I would assist her with the difficult day-to-day problems she was having. We worked together to overcome those problems and that Healthcare Training Center increased revenue by 100 percent! The owner had to rent out another building just to provide space for all the new students and programs.

My education, skills and experience over the last 27 years have afforded me the opportunity to become an expert at what I do. There are thousands of healthcare providers and business owners in need of my services. Thanks to my dedication, hard work and persistence, I am able to give back to my community and turn a profit

If anyone is interested in becoming a Nurse Entrepreneur, you can and should do it. The world is changing and this is your opportunity to achieve financial freedom. Like I did more than two decades ago, you have to make a conscientious decision to improve your economic situation. You must want it and be willing to work hard to make it happen. There is no question that it is hard out here but there are numerous career opportunities for an individual with a healthcare background.

RTCLNC, LLC also provides health and wellness workshops where our students design awareness products. Some examples of their work include our sickle cell and asthma products. Chase Jackson designed the sickle cell product and Jordan Jackson designed the Asthma product. The two young men are wellness coaches at RTCLNC, LLC Healthcare Solutions. All Rights Reserved.

BULLY ME NO MORE

This workshop is designed to help decrease bullying in the community by advocating appropriate social skills and build self-esteem by helping victims find a voice. Our youth will learn how to recognize when they are being bullied and how they should respond if this happens to them. The workshop provides activities that allow the children to role-play and practice the new social skills learned in this workshop. The children are taught to report bullying to their parents and teachers. The parents are encouraged to follow-up with the school.

MAKING HEALTHY NUTRITIONAL CHOICES

This workshop is designed to assist our youths make healthier life choices. Our health and wellness professional will provide activities that coach, motivate and inspire our youth to make healthy life and food choices. Wellness equipment, children's books, videos, and other research- based material are used to help assist the youth to identify bad habits that lead to unhealthy life choices and tips for making healthy life choices are discussed. The health and wellness programs under this umbrella include multiple health and wellness events. Healthier life choices are achieved by making healthy food choices, exercise and behavior modification.

SUBSTANCE PREVENTION PROGRAM

The Substance Prevention Program helps to create awareness needed to stop drug & gang activity in the community. The key-note speaker helps both the children and the parents to understand how gang/drug activity starts, why it continues, and what we all can do to stop our youth from becoming victims of gangs and drugs.

DIABETIC WORKSHOP

RTCLNC, LLC diabetic workshop is for people diagnosed with diabetes. The group meets every month year round and provides support, education, counseling, contact with area professionals for consultation purposes. Participants learn to manage their conditions and thrive in their daily lives in an environment that promotes camaraderie. RTCLNC, LLC staff participate as program planners and presenters.

TOBACCO CESSATION WORKSHOP

This workshop is designed to assist smokers that are motivated to stop smoking. Sandra Anderson is the speaker and provides the necessary tools to help our clients identify smoking triggers and provide support for the participants to cope with the triggers. Participants learn how to change their behavior and stay motivated to quit smoking.

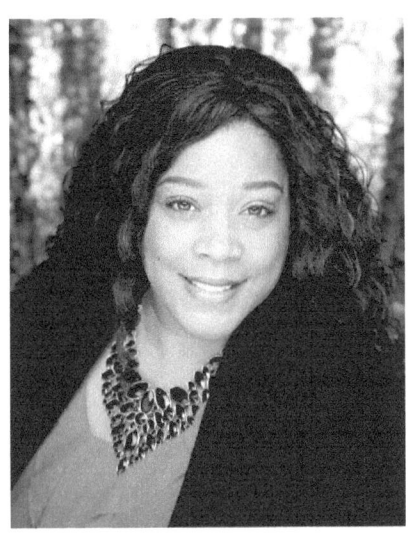

About The Author

Professor Renalda T. Carter, MSN, RN is the Founder and Senior Consultant for RTC Legal Nurse Consulting. Ms. Carter has over 27 years of experience in the healthcare field. She is also currently the Professor of Healthcare Law and Ethics at Harris-Stowe State University Anheuser-Bush School of Business. Ms. Carter obtained both her Bachelor and Master degrees in Nursing and Nursing Administration from the University of Missouri-St. Louis. She is nationally known for providing healthcare consulting services, motivational speaking, and as a healthcare educator. If you are an attorney, a healthcare provider or own a Healthcare Training Center and need assistance with providing healthcare training, medical litigation or growing your healthcare training business, contact

Professor Carter on Linked-In. She can also be reached at her virtual office on Facebook at RTCLNC, LLC Healthcare Solutions. "There is a better way!"

To Contact The Author:

https://www.facebook.com/RTCHealthcareSolutions/

https://www.linkedin.com/in/professor-renalda-carter-07771821

From RN to CEO
CHANGING LANES

BY

Venus Ricks, RN

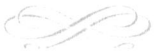

The journey to becoming a Nursepreneur began far before I was an actual Nurse. The road I traveled was long, often empty, and had many detours. Understanding the dynamics of my past and present circumstances was encouraging enough for me to attempt to break the family cycle of substance and alcohol abuse as well as incarceration. I was determined to create a new legacy for my children and eventually grandchildren that would include accomplishments versus failures. I understood for that to be possible, I had to be honest with myself, identifying barriers that could prevent me from accomplishing my goal.

I was the product of teenage parents, both were incarcerated during my early childhood years and had heroin addictions. I grew up in a family that believed that "street hustling" was as legal as going to a 9 to 5 job. My family was faithful, loyal, and dedicated to the fast life. I knew what that meant… especially for me. I clearly understood it meant I had to work extra hard to achieve the basic accomplishments. Those basic accomplishments like finishing high school and getting a job would require self-dedication and self-motivation because the odds were stacked against me. I knew I had to beat those odds and not let the odds beat me. But how??? It was hard, very hard. It's always easier to follow the crowd, fit in, or live up to the expectations of family or the statistical analysis of society. The only way to beat this was CHANGE. I had to be different. Better. But how? How can you change when everything around is the same? How do you go left when everyone is going right? This was a question I kept asking myself. It wasn't until I was arrested at the age 23 for stealing at an amusement park in Los Angeles, California that I received an answer to my question. That was the defining moment in my life.

Sitting in a jail cell thousands of miles away from my 2-½ year-old son, I felt like a failure. I had failed my son. I let him down. I began to reflect on the visits I had at the prison with my mom and I began to cry because I realized I had done to my son exactly what my parents did to me and I hated myself for it! It was in that moment that I CHANGED my life and answered my own question. I prayed to GOD, asking for his mercy to get me out of the situation and back to my son. I told GOD if he allowed me to return to my hometown of Baltimore, back to the arms of my son, I promised obedience and change. He answered my prayers and I CHANGED! My thoughts changed, my actions changed, my priorities changed. It was the hardest process ever. I began looking for jobs, eventually finding a position through a temp agency. In 1997, I began working as a temporary medical biller. This is when I developed a desire for the medical field. The assignment ended early in the spring of 1998. At that time, I was a single mother with an African American son. Understanding the significance of that; I knew, for his sake, I had to find a field where I could gain and keep steady employment. I was proficient as a medical biller, but knew I needed more training to land a position in the medical field; therefore, I began searching for a training programs that offered a Medical Billing program. I found and enrolled into the Medix School in Towson, MD. Medix offered various healthcare training programs such as Medical Office Assistant (front office), Medical Assisting (front and back office), and Dental Assistant. My plan was to enroll in the Medical Office Assistant Program; however, one of the Enrollment Specialists encouraged me to go for Medical Assisting because it consisted of both the front office and back office training.

I took the Enrollment Specialist's advice. Although I was skeptical, I enrolled in the 10-month program. That was the beginning of a major life change for me. By the time school started in August, I was pregnant with my second child. At this point, it became imperative that I completed this program. I was excited and optimistic about my new career choice, but at the same time scared and pessimistic. I knew I faced challenges that could prevent me from completing this program. Here I was a young black girl; who was 23, unmarried, with one child, and another on the way. I faced the challenge of being an inner city black female living in a subsidized apartment in one of the roughest neighborhoods in the city. I have always faced but fought through tribulations like the feeling of not being good or smart enough. I've encountered those things all my life. You see, when your mom and dad were incarcerated during your trust and confidence building years, you grow up having moments of uncertainty but you learn to push through, so that's what I did.

During my first week of school, those challenges presented themselves in full force. My car broke down, which meant I now had to use public transportation to get to school. I lived in the city and the program was in the county. As the pressure and stress piled on, my two faithful friends showed up. Throughout my life, I have had two friends who would show up whenever something went wrong. Their names are Doubt and Uncertainty and here they were; they told me it was impossible. Quit, they said! How are you going to do it? How are you going to get to Towson, MD every day, get your son to day care, and get to school on time with no car? I was ready to quit, but I didn't. I made the decision to utilize public transportation and do what needed to be done for my son and me. I found out which Light Rail trains and buses I needed to utilize to continue school. I was so glad I did. I totally loved school and everything about it! I loved being hands on and the interactions I had with my classmates. I loved making people feel better and I loved the way it made me feel! This was it! I found my niche! This was my CHANGE agent!!

During the Christmas break (New Year's Eve), I went into preterm labor and had a baby girl. Eager to finish with my starting cohorts, as soon as I got the green light from my Obstetrician, I went back to school. I was excited about being back in school, but scared and nervous because I had a premature newborn baby at home. I couldn't concentrate. I began to think, maybe I returned too quickly. This presented new a challenge for me. I began to be depressed about leaving my baby girl. She was premature and so fragile. I had to reassure myself this was the appropriate thing to do because my kids would be the beneficiaries of this training. I moved forward, but it wouldn't prevent me from worrying or having periods of anxiety about leaving her for the hours I was in school. I began to question my motherly skills and abilities. I would ask myself, "Am I a good mother? Why did I rush back so fast? Will she be ok?"

My grandmother babysat. She helped by staying with me during the week and going home on the weekends so I didn't have to travel with my baby in the cold; however, there was a major issue with that arrangement. As much as I loved my grandmother and she loved me and my children, I knew she was an alcoholic. Although she promised to refrain from drinking while she babysat, I felt terrible; but my choices were limited. So, I prayed and kept going. I completed my program in the summer of 1999, five weeks after my starting classmates because of the delivery. But I did it! It felt so good because once again I overcame my challenges.

After graduating, I was offered a position at the local City Health Department on their mobile health van as a Laboratory Technician/Phlebotomist, providing HIV/Syphilis testing and education to under-privileged and under-served communities. You couldn't tell me nothing!! The Health Department?! I was so excited, but again came challenges. Was I good enough? This was my first job as a phlebotomist!! I was scared. I knew I would be working with a unique population, IV drug user, young adults, etc. I knew this population wasn't tolerable of being stuck multiple times, so I better had known what I was doing!! I rolled my sleeves up and jumped right in and, with some minor mistakes, I overcame that challenge which groomed me to be become one of the best phlebotomists in the city. I knew if I could handle this population ,I was ready to further my career. This was the beginning of a burning desire to become a Registered Nurse.

Thereafter, I started taking classes at the Community College. I was only able to take two classes per semester for a while because I was a full-time mother and a full-time employee; therefore, it took longer than usual to complete the task, but I was determined to achieve my dreams. That is, to become an RN. While matriculating through the process, I worked various full and part-time jobs in the healthcare profession to support my children and myself. For the first time in my life, I had choices and options. I enjoyed my tenure at the Health Department. I learned a great deal attending conferences, trainings and seminars focused on the various STD's, but was I ready to move on.

    I eventually left the Healthcare Department, adding to my resume Clinical Research Associate. I landed a position at a Pharmaceutical Clinical Trial Company, learning the research side of the healthcare industry. This position empowered me; it required professionalism. I could no longer show up for work five minutes late without consequences or call out at the last minute without being written up; it made me accountable for my actions. It required more of me and my skills, knowledge, and abilities. I realized it was an opportunity for me to improve and get better. I loved my job at the Health Department but it didn't require me to do better; therefore, I was not being my best self.

    But this better came with a price. This company micromanaged their employees and I hated it. I hated the way they treated their employees. I hated not having flexibility or freedom in my life. But I had to work to provide for my kids. I thought I could find better so I ended up leaving this company to work for a Japanese pharmaceutical Clinical Trial company. They had better pay, a newer facility, and more opportunity for growth but the same morale. There was no appreciation of the employees and family was expected to be secondary to the job. It was while working here that it became clear to me I needed to eventually own my own business if I wanted to have flexibility and the freedom to prioritize things in my life. I had no clue how I was going to have my own business. At that time, it wasn't possible. My thought process was, "I'm only a phlebotomist, how am I going to make this happen?" At this point, I had mastered coming up with a master plan (when I needed one) so that's what I did.

I wanted to pursue school on a full-time basis, but I needed a position that allowed me flexibility; so, I used previous job skills to grandfather myself in as a CNA through the Maryland Board of Nursing. I knew once I became a CNA, I could use my phlebotomy skills along with my CNA certification to work in various settings. I landed a position in the Emergency Room as a ER Tech while working in various hospitals as agency CNA and pursing school full-time. Although the agency positions were flexible, they did not offer health insurance often. My husband was a contractor truck driver; therefore, he did not receive benefits. We needed health insurance, so I had to find a part-time, benefited position. I searched and was fortunate to find a phlebotomy position at the local community hospital, Good Sam, performing AM draws. The position consisted of me going to various nursing homes to draw their morning labs from their patients. I enjoyed the AM draws. I had benefits and it was flexible. It was the perfect job.

While working at Good Sam, the hospital offered their employees an opportunity to enroll in their LPN (License Practical Nurse) Program through a collaboration with the Community College. This was perfect because it offered another way for me to reach my goal of becoming an RN, especially since I had recently applied but wasn't accepted. I was already a student at the college, so I applied and was offered a seat in the upcoming program. I started the program in the summer of 2007. Because of the demands of school, I had to transfer from the Outpatient Phlebotomy position to an Inpatient Laboratory Processer, where I received lab specimen, such as blood and urine, and processed them for testing. Things were going well. I could then keep up with the demands from school and completed in 2008.

Upon completing my studies and passing the NCLEX, I was ready to move on to the next phase in my career. I was proud of myself because I had overcome many obstacles to get here, but it was worth. I began looking for LPN positions. My current employer had positions open on their acute care units. I interviewed and was hired as an LPN on a Med-Surg/Oncology Unit. The roles of LPNs had changed tremendously during this time. There weren't many of them working in acute care settings. The RNs were not happy when they worked with me or behind me because I had limited functions, which meant more work for them. I often felt inadequate as if I was not a real nurse. They made me feel bad about being a LPN. It wasn't a good feeling, but it pushed me to want more. I realize the uncomfortable spot was motivating me. It made work harder and strive for the next level. I knew the next level was to become a RN.

After being an LPN for a year, I enrolled in the LPN to RN bridge program. I knew this decision would get me one step closer to my goal of owning my own business. My job agreed to pay for it but I couldn't work part-time this time, which meant I had to work as a full-time LPN and attend school full-time - not to mention the school was a 45-minute drive. I knew it would be challenging, but I also knew it was possible. With every obstacle I overcame, it helped me build confidence instead of fear. I began to realize my thoughts shaped my actions and I only could accomplish things I believed I could. Likewise, if I believed I couldn't accomplish something, I wouldn't. Understanding this concept helped me to become much more positive and believe in myself much more than I ever had.

I discovered the nursing field was an excellent opportunity for me to change the dynamics of my family's life and mine. I also knew it would help me get to my goal of owning my own business. I was ready to move forward. I completed and graduated the LPN to RN Bridge Program. This was a bittersweet moment for me because the lady who raised me wasn't there to celebrate my accomplishment for the first time in my life. My grandmother, the one person who never let me down, had passed away. I was an emotional wreck at my graduation. The only remedy for my pain was to make her very proud of me.

Once I graduated and completed the RN-NCLEX, I continued to work on the same unit at Good Samaritan hospital as an RN. I had more autonomy as an RN, but the workload remained the same. I wanted more, so I joined the Research Council with hopes of getting what I was looking for. I didn't get it. I found myself feeling like a robot, giving medicine room to room. I did not feel I was utilizing my skills and knowledge to reach my full potential. I tried to transfer to the ER Department, but was unable to because I didn't have critical care experience. I then tapped into my desire to work in the research side of the field and began to search job opportunities, applying for multiple positions on USA Jobs.

My first response was from National Institute of Health (NIH). I couldn't believe it! NIH was my dream job. They called me for an interview and I was granted a federal position as a Clinical Research Nurse. I absolutely couldn't believe it; this was a dream come true! I would have never thought this was possible. Me, Venus Ricks! I'm the little girl whose parents were both in prison by the time she was five years old; the angry little girl who wanted to fight all the time. The young lady who dropped out of school, graduating from an alternative school, and was arrested for stealing. And that's when it hit me. I had overcome all these obstacles.

I was ecstatic, but then I got scared. The job required me to have a security clearance, which meant I had to do a financial and security background check. I was ok with the financial check, but a background check! My friends Fear and Doubt came to see me as usual. I just knew my past would haunt me!! I had to get myself together. This wasn't the time for negativity. If I was going to pass this security clearance, I had to believe that I would; so I did. I proceeded with transparency and disclosed the arrest, praying and hoping it wouldn't be held against me. I got the job! This was major for me! Applying and getting this position was a huge turning point in my life because I never thought this was possible. This job opened doors in my mind and thus, began opening doors in my life.

I had never been through a rigorous process like this; the interview was 4 hours. I studied for the interview and prepped by updating myself on what I already knew about research. I researched information on NIH and the facility from which I would be working. I researched interviewing questions. This was all done to be prepared as much as I could and it worked! I was officially a Federal Research Nurse at one of the most influential healthcare facilities in the world. The irony of this is that the center I would be working at was NIDA (National Institutes of Drug and Alcohol). Both drugs and alcohol had negatively affected my childhood so this was an honor. Understanding the effects of both I thought would help me heal my internal wounds for my childhood. I realized I had broken a barrier in my life as I crossed into another chapter. With hard work and perseverance, I could accomplish anything.

While working at NIH, I began to pursue other opportunities for Nurses. I was encouraged by my Aunt Shug to take a Delegating Nurse course. She had an Assisted Living facility and her current Delegating Nurse was about to retire. She wanted me to replace her when she retired. I took the training and began Delegating for my aunt; this was the beginning of my Nursepreneur journey. My position at NIH wasn't living up to my expectations. I had gone from working in a 12-hour a day, fast pace Med-Surg/Oncology unit to a very slow pace, hardly not doing anything environment. I was also experiencing workplace issues that made me very uncomfortable. I began to realize I didn't like it as much as I thought I would.

While working at NIH, I also worked part-time as a weekend Charge Nurse for the Department of Public Safety and Correctional Services (DPSCSC). The Regional Manager offered me a position as the Assistant Director of Nursing (ADON) for Pre-Trial Division. I was happy, but was unsure about taking the position. I had reservations because working in corrections had many challenges, especially as an Administrator. After thinking and rethinking multiple times, I accepted. I realized this was an opportunity for me to get some administration experience. I was honored because I didn't apply for the position, which meant I was being recognized for my work performance. I was excited about my new position, but didn't let it stop me from pursuing my dreams of becoming an entrepreneur and business owner. I continued to work as a Delegating Nurse with opportunities to add on other facilities.

During this time, I was learning the Assisted Living industry and began to realize the need for services and training that would increase resident safety and staff knowledge; as a result, I opened Vital Sign Nursing and Training. While working for DPSCS, I pursued other healthcare training courses that would enhance my Delegating Nurse and training role. I began to contract out my expertise and training services to other Assisted Living facilities. My Delegating Nurse experience increased my awareness of abuse of vulnerable adults and I didn't like it at all. It was this experience that motivated me to eventually open my very own Assisted Living facility. This also served as my motivation to leave DPSCS due to the inability to get along with their leadership. I had experienced many ethical dilemmas during my tenure as ADON. I didn't feel comfortable anymore; it was time for me to leave.

This was a rough time for me because it was difficult finding a position that would pay me the salary I needed to support my kids. My husband and I were separated, my daughter's school tuition was $20,000/year, and my son was recently acquitted of a criminal matter where I had spent all my saving on his attorney's fee. I found myself in a very dark place. I was broke and depressed. My main priority was to focus on my daughter's education; she had worked very hard to be accepted into an Ivy League prep school and I wasn't going to jeopardize that. It was at that moment I realize I could not work in corporate America anymore. I wanted freedom.

Freedom to control my own life. I knew corporate America wouldn't give me what I wanted, so I had to give it to myself.

I stopped looking for good paying positions and accepted a position at Mount Washington Elementary and Middle School as a School Nurse in Baltimore City. It was a significant decrease in pay but it gave me what I wanted – FREEDOM - freedom to make the decisions that are important in my life and pursue my career and personal goals. No, I wasn't making money, but I was making history with this job. This job afforded me the ability to get my daughter to school and time to plan my future endeavors. I faced difficulties from the very beginning. It was always a struggle, but I was always determined.

I researched all the rules and regulations applicable to assisted living facilities. I began to vision how my facility would look. I had a major problem though; I didn't have much money! How was I going to make this happen with limited financial resources? I started thinking and my best friend popped up in my head! She had healthcare experience, she knew this industry well, and she had money so I asked her to partner with me. She agreed! Happy, excited, and anxious all at the same time, we began looking for homes that would accommodate our vision. I had this vision of a spacious, well-lit home-style environment, but it was hard finding a house that fit my vision. I kept looking and looking with no luck. Eventually, I began to get discouraged; but while looking on Zillow one day, I saw a picture of a house captioned, "Perfect for an Assisted Living". I clicked on the picture and instantly knew this house was it. I scheduled an appointment for a viewing, and my best friend and I both loved it. We sealed the deal on the spot. We agreed to share the financial responsibilities 50/50. I was ready and she was ready so I thought. However, my best friend pulled out. I was devastated; how she could she? It was over. My dreams were shot down just like that. Once again someone else controlled my destiny and I couldn't let this happen.

Again, I had to think of a master plan. How was I going to make this work? I went to the landlord and asked if he could work with me. I promised him if he gave me a chance, I wouldn't let him down. It worked and he agreed to help me!! I spent every dollar I had and every dollar I earned on this project. I searched for bargains, purchased some things on credit, and received donated furniture from a large assisted living community. I prayed and prayed and prayed; I knew the only person that could help get me through this was GOD. That's who I talked to several times a day and depended on. GOD was coming through for me. My request for trainings were increasing and I was making enough money to help fund my project and pay my bills. My dreams were coming to life.

Having been raised by a loving grandmother, Mable Anthony Stokes, who in her everyday living exemplified her love and concern for people in her community, I was motivated to name my facility, **"MABLE'S HOUSE".** I had birthed another child "Mable's House" a home like environment where those vulnerable adults were truly treated as family, their dignity was respected, and they were given a sense a genuine security and safety. I was ready to open. I recruited my sister-in-law and another best friend to be my mangers. I submitted my application and waited for the response. The overseeing agency, Office of Healthcare Quality (OHCQ), called with a date. My team and I were ready.

The surveyor came out; we were prepared or so we thought. The house had a beautifully built balcony on the upper portion of the house, but the surveyor had issues with the height of the balcony, which she did not believe was in compliance with the zonings code particular to the American with Disabilities (ADA). Her suggestion was to tear down the deck and rebuild it. Rebuild? I couldn't believe what I was hearing. It wasn't possible for the balcony to be rebuilt; I couldn't financially support that. My anxiety level had elevated tremendously, but I had to remain calm. I had another option; she could request for an environmentalist to come out to inspect the balcony. That was the option I chose. Of course, I was worried because I knew if the environmentalist agreed with the surveyor, it was over because I absolutely did not have the money to rebuild the balcony. The environmentalist took forever to come out but when he did, I was cleared!! I could breathe again. I had been holding my breath for about three weeks. I received my licensed and opened.

My grand opening was wonderful. I invited Friends, Family, Social Workers, Nurses, and the Community. I was licensed for eight beds. I just knew my beds would be filled in two months' tops, but I faced difficulties filling those beds. It was more difficult than I imagined. Being a Registered Nurse, I just knew once I opened the beds would fill up immediately. I admitted one resident in two months. I was worried because the bills associated with the facility were piling in; however, I stayed the course, remain dedicated, and persevered. I believed in my dream and my ability to succeed. I began to re-strategize, focusing on marketing. I began with LOGO development, business cards, and brochures. I went to the hospital where my nursing career started, other community hospitals, rehab centers, and long term care facilities. Social Workers, Case Managers, and Referral Agents were all on my radar. I knew I had to be persistent, so I continuously networked.

A big break came through when my stepmother had set an appointment for a vendor presentation. This was huge! One of the local community hospitals had agreed to allow me to present to their Social Work Department to become one of their Assisted Living vendors. YES!!! I went professionally dressed; ordered pizzas, salads, and drinks for them; and arrived 20 minutes early, only to be told they cancelled the meeting because the census was high. Disappointed, angry, and depressed were the emotions I felt. Although I was upset, I agreed to come back next month. So, next month, I did the exact same thing and so did they - CANCELLED again!! I'm like, are you serious? Now I'm mad! Why would they have me come all the way here without cancelling prior to the appointment? Again ,the director asked if I could come back next month. At this point, I'm about to have nervous breakdown because my funds were getting very low. I had anticipated all the beds were going to be filled by now. The bills were steady coming and I was running out of funds. I was finally able to admit a second resident; however, I had hired someone for day shift so I would be available to do marketing during the day since I worked the night shift.

Eventually, I had to borrow money from my sister to keep operations going. I verbally agreed to return to the hospital, but in mind I'm telling myself I'm not coming back here. As I began to walk to my car something hit me. I realized I was giving up; failing and failure wasn't an option. I asked myself how you can quit after coming this far? How do you expect to be a vendor if you don't return? My positive self overpowered my negative self and I returned to the hospital the next month, presented my services, and nailed it!! I did it! I was now a vendor. They could officially refer patients to my facility. They were very impressed with my determination and dedication and immediately started referring patients. I filled my beds in eight weeks. My entrepreneurship journey was defined by this moment. Failure was so close I could kiss it, but opportunity was even closer. I just had to choose one.

Once I chose opportunity, opportunities chose me. Doors began to open one after another. All I had to do was walk through them. Vital Sign Nursing and Training added on additional training courses and consulting services with expanding goals. I have since partnered up to open PHO-VITAL SIGN HOME CARE, a Residential Services Agency having two clients in summer of 2016 and now having 40+ clients and growing. Mabel's House Assisted Living now has a second location. It is unreal what I have accomplished in three years; however, what is even more amazing is that I'm just getting started. What lies ahead is up to me. I now know accomplishments are a matter of the mind, and I always keep that in mind when it really matters. The greatest reward of all is acknowledging that the more I help others, the greater impact it has on my own life.

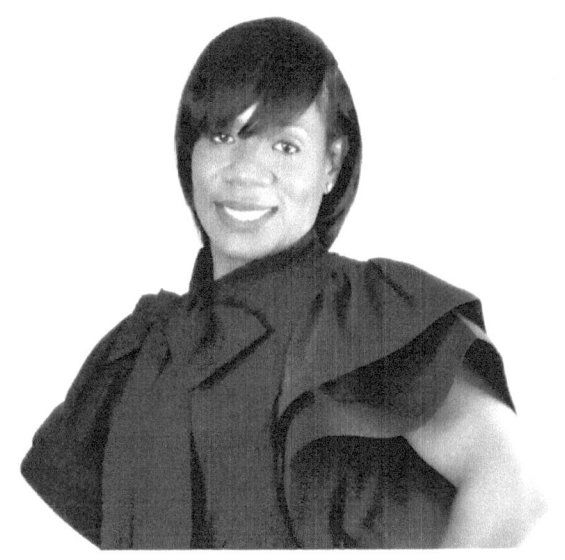

About the Author

Venus Ricks, RN - CEO/Founder of Vital Sign Nursing and Training turned her passion into profit. Her love for people and desire to help others is why she became a Nurse. As a Registered Nurse, Venus took her nursing experience beyond the hospital floors. Inspired by her own story and desire to help others, she launched her healthcare training center. Ambitious at heart, never letting any grass grow under her feet, she didn't stop at training. Her tenure as a Delegating Nurse and need, motivated her to open Mabel's House Assisted Living in honor of her grandmother Mabel, serving the elderly and vulnerable population. Simultaneously, Pho-Vital Sign Home Care was also launched, serving the same population. She takes pride in overcoming obstacles and never giving up, which has allowed her to obtain a level of success in healthcare.

To Contact The Author:

www.vitalsignnursing.com

vitalsignnursing@gmail.com

IG: vital_sign_nursing

FB: facebook.com/venusricks & facebook.com/vitalsignnursingtraining

THE NURSE ENTREPRENEUR COLLECTIVE

BY
Michelle G. Rhodes MHS, RN

HOW IT ALL STARTED

Even as a young girl I used to love to help people. Little Michelle was always the one taking in the groceries for mom, making cookies with my grandmother, or helping someone change a bandage. It was just in me to be helpful, to ask "why" toward multiple questions. I guess you could say that I was an inquisitive child.

While going through high school, I found a new love in studying the human body. You see, my inclination towards the love of science took me through school with high marks (A's and B's) as well as a love for anatomy and physiology. The way that the human formed and worked together to function, simply captivated me.

By high school graduation, I knew that whatever it was that I decided to do, it would include a Health and Wellness component. After whittling down my college majors to Nursing or Pharmacy, I discovered that Physics would be needed for Pharmacy as a major, which eliminated that choice, right there for me.

I was definitely NOT one that enjoyed Physics, and I discovered that Nursing was my true calling, as I loved being there for others when they needed me the most. I poured my heart and soul into studying and thus Nursing was my career choice. Fast forward to graduating Magna Cum Laude from

Florida Agricultural and Mechanical University in the Fall of 1995, and then a Masters of Health Sciences in 2001 from the University of Central Florida. I enjoyed working in the business of healthcare and the Insurance industry afforded me the opportunity to do that as a Nurse. I found a good rhythm of in case management, medical case management, and population health care management. I truly enjoy the combination of health and business and this love has carried me through my 21-year career. But last November "IT" happened! Symptoms of burnout appeared and the strong desire for the "next level" took root and I was no longer happy. I begin to think to myself, is this all there is and will I do this until age 65? Will I be crunching numbers and helping companies save money for another 20 years? I knew the answer was NO and I was ready. I was beyond ready to be a Nurse entrepreneur and had been slowly preparing for it over the years. You see I had been setting aside savings monthly for this moment. By combining my love for business, health and coaching others, I rolled all of this up into my passion. You see I had become a Certified Mentor back in 2004, as well as a Coach with Wellcoaches back in 2009. I had helped my husband start up his business after he retired from the Military.

MY TRANSITION

Up until that point you November I had no idea how to package up all of these experiences and formulate it into what I love to do most. But it was almost like the Lord shined HIS light on my soul and showed me with clarity what I needed to do. You see I realized, after talking to so many Nurses over the years I found it to be a problem that we knew how to care for another human being that may or may not be on deaths' doorstep, but have very little information as how to wrap up that specialized knowledge and market themselves. Most Nurses never realize that in reality we became Entrepreneurs the day that we earned this license. Once I realized that for myself, my path towards Nurse entrepreneurship had begun.

I immediately hired a coach who was completely available for me and who would get me on the fastest track to sharing my passion with the world. She knew immediately that I was fully ready to help others. She was a woman of excellence, positivity and spirituality. With her straightforward guidance, I have pinned my first book, "RNTERPRISE" and this book serves as number two and is just the beginning for me. My long-term goal is to have my writings serves as the backbone to Nurse Entrepreneurship electives in Nursing Programs across the country.

THE BURNING QUESTION

Why is that this type of information is not readily available to Nurses across the country, was my initial thought? We as Nurses should be prepared to have this as a career option as soon as we graduate. There are so many companies and corporations out there who could benefit from our specialized knowledge. Thinking to myself, this information is so valuable, why do we have to go out and learn it ourselves? It is understood that there are key concepts and a core knowledge base that all Nurses need in order to perform and for programs to be accredited. With 60% of the Nurses showing the signs of burn out at any given time (Cimiotti, J., et al., 2012). we must find a better way to make these caregivers happy. If 20% (1) of Nurses are leaving the career after just serving two years, why isn't someone out there trying to do something about that startling statistic? Education is too costly and timely to just throw away after pouring large amounts of time and money into obtaining this degree and licensure. Not to mention the skill set alone. It is up to us to wrap up this knowledge and serve the people or organizations that need us in different ways and healthcare, not just at the bedside. There are home healthcare agencies, assisted living facilities, Nurse educators, and Nurse consultants that need our help everywhere across the world. These facts deserve a second chance, and my honest opinion a viable solution. As with any starting point, this research helped me to formulate my burning question that needed to be answered. "Why isn't this entrepreneurial education available to Nurses much sooner, rather them later?" This is what began my quest of coaching Nurses from where they are, to where they want to be in business. Many of us have backgrounds that are suitable to qualify as us an expert, but go under- utilized, through no fault of our own.

BUILD YOUR RNTERPRISE

Now serving as a Coach for Nurses who want to start their own businesses, I delight myself in sharing what I've learned with them. My ultimate goal is to get this knowledge into the hands of a local community college or even universities to add this information as a noncredit elective and a nursing programs across the country. We all should know how to start a business, how to wrap up our knowledge and market ourselves to those out there who need it the most. As I have always told my clients, there are many companies out there that will pay for your knowledge and skill. If the market does not know about you, how can they find you for help?

I encourage you today to wrap up everything that you know and formulate it into entrepreneurship. The risk definitely outweighs the benefits, as who else will pay you to work your own schedule at your own leisure? Will pay the maximum rate of your worth? Who will pay you maximum rate for everything that you know? Who will employ for your passion? No one but you. You hold all of the answers in the palm hand, heart and brain, so let's get to it! *Find your passion, get some help from a mentor, identify your target market, write a business plan, get some help with your branding and marketing and share your message with the world*!

Let's discuss these steps in a little more detail.

Mentoring and Passion. These are a few of the things that I use in coaching my clients as my business move them from employee to entrepreneur. It's always a good advice and brave step to hire a **coach or mentor** in the early stages. That person can help you avoid pitfalls and making mistakes that they may have learned from in the past. This will save you time and energy. They also will save you money in the long run as you have not wasted it on countless mistakes. Next you want to develop your passion. Find out what it is that makes you happy, that makes you great, and that you love so much you would do it for free if you could! Your love for your passion will carry you through the hard times, and when there are times when you feel like giving up. As with anything there are ups and downs and there are bound to be times where you want to throw in the towel. These are just a few of the awesome benefits to having a mentor and identifying your passion.

Let's talk next about identifying your *target market*. You see, identify the specific persons that you are targeting for your services is a key element of success when becoming an entrepreneur. A business cannot truly market to everyone, they know their ideal customer like the back of their hands. They have done the research and are prepared to offer a specific service or product to a specific type of individual. So, when thinking about what you are offering to the marketplace, please consider the ideal person who is purchasing from you. How do they look? How much money do they make? Where do they shop? What do they like? What is their family structure like? How old are they? Does gender matter? What do they enjoy? What are their hobbies? How are they benefit from your product or service? These are all things that one has to answer so that the marketing can be targeted specifically to that group of individuals. Only then will you experience success because you know exactly who you were targeting and your marketing.

Moving onto the bigger piece of the puzzle of start-up is *business planning*. This might require some major assistance if you have never gone into business before. At this stage, you should get legal by filing all paperwork with your state, and applying for state and local taxes if you have to. You might even need to obtain certain permits as well. Now that you're ready, the business plan will include certain steps depending on how big your business will be. This all varies based on if you will need financing or if you will be applying for a small business loan along the way. If you are a solo entrepreneur you might not require a big business plan as if you were going to ask for business loans. At the very least you could do a S.W.O.T. analysis to see where you live in the way of your skills and strengths, weaknesses, opportunities and threats. This business plan sometimes is a very large document, and is why I stated that you might need to get a little assistance. Your executive summary, will give a snapshot of your business. The organization and management section will tell how your business will be overseen. Next is any funding requests and why. You will then give a brief description of your company, what you do and why. Be sure to show and illustrate what makes you different from others. The product line or service line demonstrates the specific products and services that you offer. Your financial projections come next, demonstrating your financial need in order to get started and how much you anticipate making. Backing up all of this data, is market research and a feasibility study, so make sure that you have done your homework.

Branding. If you are in entrepreneur or aspiring to become an entrepreneur, is a well-known fact that your branding speaks volumes to the ideal client in which you attempting to connect with. When they see you in the community, that's your brand. What they tell others about you, is your brand. Your mission statement, vision and values all comprise your brand. Your brand includes a promise to deliver a certain "thing". The specific and look and color scheme present on your graphic material becomes known as a part of your brand. So, today let's look at a few items that will help you become recognized as you develop your brand. It may change and evolve and that is perfectly okay. Just do not allow any of this to stop your progression.

Number one, research colors and the meaning of certain colors, these colors on your advertisements will help draw in your client. According to what type of emotions you evoke through the color schemes that you use on your website, cards, and marketing materials, they will feel a certain way when they see your brand. Your customers should enjoy this feeling, and that is why they follow your brand and purchase your product or services. What type of emotions are you bringing forth in your ideal client?

Number two, make sure that all photography of you, your events, your products, and even your logo is done professionally. Do not skip out on this piece. Although it seems like a small thing, your presentation is everything. If you cut corners here, your customer base will know it and recognize it.

The customer may feel like you might cut corners and other areas of business. They might start to think negatively about your brand right from the start. Do they provide the best customer service? Do they return calls in a timely manner? Are they exhibiting a bad reputation when it comes to your pricing? Are they really trying to give me the best at the best price, or just be cheap all around? Let your first impression be your best impression! Leave no room for doubt concerning your brand.

Number three take a look at everything that you've done to make yourself stand out in the marketplace. How are you different? How are you perceived? Do you blend in with all of the rest competition? You see, in any business there is competition everywhere, so you will have to put a twist on your brand that will make you stand out from the ordinary. No matter what type of business, or what line of service that you provide, there will always be someone else out there attempting to do it better. But do you know what? Only you can do it your way! So, shine brightly, and let the world see who you are! Be bold, be fierce, be you! These Branding 101 tips entails just a few items of creating your signature stamp, but you will definitely be on your way if you implement these few suggestions!

Marketing. When it comes to marketing, you must start with a plan. Trust me - marketing can turn into a black hole that you just toss money into if you don't go in with a strategy. There are so many marketing opportunities available these days, and any of them sounds like the next greatest idea, but not all are right for your business and for talking to YOUR client. That's why it's imperative to create a marketing plan, both when you're first starting your business and at the start of every year.

Your first marketing plan is going to be a lot of guessing. You're going to try things, and if they don't provide the desired results, that just means it's time to adjust your plan. As you try different marketing tactics and measure the results, you'll have more to go on as you move forward. Starting out, it will be all trial and error. The important part is that you have a plan from which to start and that you continuously measure your results; this will go a long way in helping you to shape a future that you desire.

If you can answer these three questions, you'll have the framework for all that comes after. Without these answers, you're literally going to be shooting in the dark. We've touched on these concepts in previous chapters, but these are things that are imperative to know when setting up your marketing plan.

1. A clear, focused reason as to why your customer will use you. We've been through this before, but what is the core reason that a customer specifically needs your services? Is it because you are so efficient? Are you more attentive, always available, an expert in one particular area?

2. Who is your target customer? Now that you know what exactly you provide, determine who the person is who needs exactly that. Write a description of that person, their likes, dislikes, age, circumstances, gender, location, etc. It might help to give this person a name. Have them in mind whenever you're creating marketing materials. Be authentic and this will resonate with your audience.

3. When it comes to this target audience, what other competitors are vying for their attention? There is always another way your target audience can spend their money. There's always another service or product that they might purchase instead. Take the time to find out what these are in your industry so that you can adapt your marketing efforts to be the better solution. Just remember that it's impossible to be better if you don't know what your competition is doing.

All of these answers come together to form your tagline, or USP (unique selling proposition). It's basically a concise version of your elevator speech. But from here, we can start to get a sense of where to focus your marketing efforts.

You might have to obtain assistance in this area as it can be a full- time job marketing your brand as well.

Your website, email listing, social media platforms, blog, podcasts etc., all hold the potential to market your products and services extremely well. Make a Marketing calendar and stick to it! Now share your message with the world, keep track on what efforts works and what doesn't, and remember **sales** ARE the key to success!

The hardest part of starting any business is the fact that, often, you're doing it alone. You can find the answer to almost any question online, but it's difficult to differentiate between what's good and what's sub-par. It's also pretty common to find conflicting information. How can you tell what's right for you and your circumstances? How can you avoid the cookie-cutter answer that might not exactly fit your situation? There is definitely something to be said for having a real person to talk to when questions arise or problems surface.

If you research the most successful people in the world, you'll see that they all had mentors. Maya Angelou mentored Oprah. Steve Jobs mentored Mark Zuckerberg. Ray Charles mentored Quincy Jones. Basically, if they are famous enough that you know their name, they probably had a mentor.

Mentors are not just people who can coach you in times of distress. They have experience, and experience is an expensive commodity. In fact, experience is the one thing that you can't buy. You can read, you can study, you can research, but there is no alternative to experience. The only way to get experience is to live through it. A mentor can provide you with business advice from the perspective of experience. In fact, having a mentor is the only real way to benefit from experience before living through it.

In addition to the general business acumen and problem solving that comes from experience, your mentor also has a network. Your mentor knows more people than you because he or she has been in the game longer. It's like moving to a new town. It would take you months or years to get to know, through experience, where to take your car to get it fixed, or which salon is the best. And you would have no cause to know certain things until you actually needed them. You would have no use in knowing which realtor to use until you were ready to purchase a home.

Similarly, a mentor has been places that you have had no need to be yet so they already know who to call for what problem. They've already dealt with situations that are, as of now, only in your future. Therefore, not only will they be able to recommend you to these resources, they will also be able to make connections that you didn't even know were possible. By having a mentor, you are leveraging an entirely different network and becoming part of it. Having a mentor is like getting a head start in business.

Also, on the surface, it might seem like the primary reason to have a mentor is to have someone to help with your questions and the problems that come up as you make your way as an entrepreneur. But that's actually the secondary reason. That reason stems from the fact that we are scared as we make our way down this path of entrepreneurship. We're scared of what we'll encounter, or that we won't do things correctly or that we'll mess up somehow. What we forget is that it is only the nuts and bolts. These things are all important and helpful, but what a mentor provides that we cannot even imagine at the outset is the grain of inspiration, the extra push of encouragement and that added bit of confidence. Having a mentor is not primarily about having someone on our side to help us see what's wrong, but with having someone in our corner who can propel us to think a little bit bigger, take a calculated risk or push ourselves outside of our comfort zone to achieve greatness.

A mentor not only knows what it takes to succeed monetarily, but also what it takes to succeed emotionally, mentally and spiritually. Decisions will undoubtedly arise down the line to which there is no right or wrong answer. It could be in regard to how best to deal with a client, or what particular path to take at a challenging business crossroad. Having a mentor in those circumstances can illuminate the course of action that is right for you as a person. The ethical dilemmas, the situations that seem to pry at your moral fiber and the job-related problems that can have big repercussions on your personal life are the instances where mentors provide the brightest light. In these instances, a mentor can be an absolute blessing.

So, having a mentor is not what people do when they can't do it themselves, or don't have the right resources. People have mentors because it opens up a new world for them, amplifies the possibilities and increases the chance for grander thought and wilder success.

Having a mentor can only increase your chance for success, and undoubtedly, will make whatever success you would've found on your own that much more expansive.

I know the nursing industry inside and out, and have mentored Nurse entrepreneurs like you, who now are thriving and living abundant lives. It fills my heart for me to see them doing what they love and being successful. I'm ready to be your mentor and to help you on your path to RNterprising. It's a wonderful experience to do what you love and to do it on your own schedule. And it's even more wonderful to watch the people who I coach go through this same transition.

It starts with just the seed of an idea and an urge to do what you love, without the unneeded stress. I've helped nurture this urge in its infancy and watched my mentees set up original, creative and successful businesses where they no longer answer to the demands of the hospital hierarchy. You can create an RNterprise that's satisfying for you AND beneficial to your clients.

Once connecting with me and completing your 90-day start up, you will also have access to my Secret Mastermind Circle (SMC). This is where mentees are placed with other business owners who might be performing in the particular type of business that you desire to run. I have connected with just a few entrepreneurs in Healthcare. The group and its representatives grow daily.

We have entrepreneurs representing the following to help you in the Mastermind:

Home Health Care Agency

Adult Day Care Center

Group Home

Nurse Travel Agency

Staffing Agency

CPR Instructors

Medicare/Medicaid Experts

Banking Representative

Non-Profit Expert

Business Plan Writer

Legal Nurse Consultant

CNA School Owner

Together, let's make your dream a reality. Let's get moving toward your success. Connect with me and, in 90 days, your dream can be well on its way to becoming reality. Once the business is started, I will continue to mentor and teach you how to build upon each one that will comprise your RNterprise. This RNterprise leads to your Legacy. Your legacy is something your family will forever be grateful that you started for years to come. These are a few steps to prepare YOU and to help you get ready to join The Nursepreneur Collective.

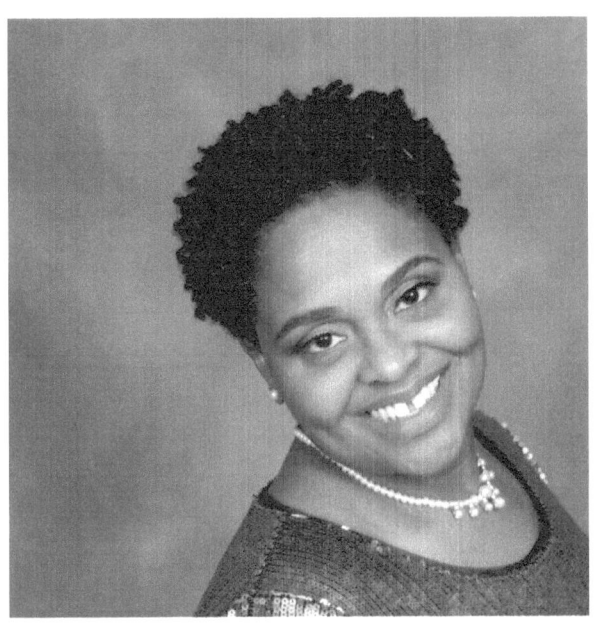

About the Author

Michelle Greene Rhodes is known as THE Life Coach and Business Consultant for Nurse Entrepreneurs. Inspired by her passion, she assists Health Professionals who struggle with the "start-up" phase of their business. She helps them free up their time, and find a purpose filled life of their own by streamlining the first steps of entrepreneurship.

Michelle graduated Nursing school at age 21 from Florida A&M University and completed graduate school at age 27 from University of Central Florida with her Masters in Health Administration. She has gone on to enjoy a 20-year career in

Nursing and has decided to enter into entrepreneurship and take a few others along the way!

Described as an intellectual and compassionate caregiver, Michelle conveys caring, empowerment and optimism in everything that she does. Many Nurses over the years have stated they learned so much from Michelle and enjoyed being around her encouraging personality.

Having become a Certified Mentor and Life Coach, she decided to immerse herself in servant leadership, giving back to those who needed the most, while starting up a business. "So many times, I had 1000 questions and very few answers," states Michelle. "I knew this was a problem that needed to be filled because, as Nurses, we are taught how to care within our specialty, but only if you're very lucky will you encounter a Veteran Nurse to help you find the answers that you need on your personal journey to entrepreneurship."

Michelle is active on all social media platforms, with avid followers.

She is an author and speaker and looks forward to releasing her first book on May 20, 2017 in Tampa, Florida, at her First Annual Health and Wealth Brunch for Health Care Professionals.

Michelle is very active in her community as an engaged and industrious member of The National Coalition of 100 Black Women as the Co-Chair of Health, and sits on the Mayors African American Advocacy Council (MAAC) in Tampa Florida.

She also is the Founder of the Tampa Chapter of Black Nurses Rock, Inc., a non-profit organization. She serves as a Certified Mentor and Wellness Coach.

She is the loving, devoted wife of retired Air Force Veteran, Albert Rhodes Jr. and a proud, loving mother of son, Jon and daughter, Ali.

Get started today and schedule time to meet with me at:

Michellerhodesonline.com for Business Coaching

IG: Instagram.com/MichelleRhodesOnline

FB: Facebook.com/MichelleRhodesOnline

WHEN NURSING ISN'T ENOUGH

BY
Jeteia L. Benson RN, MSN, FNP-C

Hello, my name is Jeteia Benson and I am a Nurse. Well, technically, I am a Nurse Practitioner, but I will get into the story shortly. I was about five years old when I told my mother I wanted to be a "baby doctor." That was right around the time my little brother was born. I helped my mother as much as possible with the baby. Helping with my brother warmed my soul, and I decided I wanted to pursue a career in healthcare. I come from the inner city, an area I could have easily become a statistic. Growing up, the odds were against me, but my family was determined to push my siblings and I to become great. The value of education and hard work was instilled in me all while growing up. Therefore, I always believed I could do anything I set my mind to.

Fast forward, I worked hard throughout high-school and was afforded the opportunity to attend the college of my choice. I chose Fisk University in Nashville, Tennessee. I excelled in college, majoring in Biology with the goal of going to medical school, or so I thought. It was not until after graduation that I realized I no longer wanted to pursue medical school.

In my opinion, I had done the worst possible thing; I had graduated from college with no direction. I had developed a love for helping the public and the spread of disease, so I decided to attend graduate school for public health. I subsequently applied and was accepted to Tulane University in New Orleans. I packed up in August 2005 and moved down to New Orleans Louisiana. I was there all of 24 hours be for we had to swiftly evacuate under the threat of a torrential storm. Hurricane Katrina happened the very next day and changed my life and path, again. After a few weeks of waiting to see how things would turn out, I landed back home in Ohio, still with no direction. I then began to find work doing other things. I worked at a microbiology lab and pharmaceutical company. After that, I worked at a charter school in the administration office before transitioning into a classroom assistant and substitute teacher role at an elementary school; all the while, I was also working as a home health aide. That was actually my first glimpse into nursing. I formed bonds with clients that I kept in touch with for years after I no longer was their caregiver.

One day, I wandered into a beauty supply store and ran into another Fiskite. She shared with me that she had once felt like I did; after graduation, she had no career direction either. She was recently accepted into a nursing program and had fallen in love. It made me wonder why I had not thought of this before, why I was working for a home care agency and did not even think to check into other healthcare options. So after our talk, I researched nursing; however, I was not convinced right away. The more I researched, the more I saw all the wonderful things Nurses do. I remembered all the kind, dedicated Nurses I had encountered throughout my life. But what really sealed the deal was the flexibility in nursing. There are literally dozens of paths for Nurses. I could be a floor Nurse, a research Nurse, a Nurse that runs clinical trials, a legal Nurse, and the list goes on. I was sold! Nursing was the field for me.

DESTINED FOR GREATNESS

In November 2007, I decided to apply for the program my Fisk sister told me about. I did not even bother looking for other programs. I was accepted and set to start an accelerated nursing program the following January. The program was a year and a half and the time whizzed by so fast I can hardly remember it.

It was now my final semester in nursing school and I was hit with a huge dilemma. I had completely run out of financial aid. I used it all between my first bachelors' degree and my nursing degree. It was Monday and I had to come up with over $5000 dollars by Friday or I would be removed from classes and dismissed from school. This was the first time I had ever experienced anything like this. I went into full-blown panic mode. Unfortunately, there was no one who could help me on such short notice. Ultimately I had no choice but to put an entire semester of tuition and fees on a credit card. I was not excited about it but did what I had to do to get over that hump. I was able to remain in my classes and complete nursing school.

August 2009 I walked across the stage and by October that year I had become a licensed Nurse. I took a job working at one of the top hospitals in the nation. Of course, I went into Pediatrics because I have always had that passion to work with children. I worked in pediatrics inpatient and outpatient until 2013. My nursing experiences was made up of Adult Cardiac Step-Down, Pediatric Cardiac Step-Down, Neonatal Intensive Care Step-Down, and General Pediatrics as a telephone triage Nurse. While working as a Registered Nurse, I also became a Nursing Clinical Instructor for one of the local colleges in Cleveland. I have always been a "teacher" deep down. As a result I still currently manage to teach at least one rotation of clinical instruction per year to do my part in educating the future Nurses of America.

While working as a floor Nurse and teaching clinical I decided it was time for me to continue furthering my career. I applied to several graduate programs and interviewed at a few only to receive rejection after rejection. While I was going through this I remember thinking, "maybe I should just give up that dream, maybe it is not meant for me." In retrospect, I am glad I did not give up because all the rejections were building my perseverance. A skill I would certainly need in all areas of life. Finally, over a year after starting to apply for graduate nursing programs I was accepted to University of Cincinnati masters program. I had a serious praise break. I also remember thinking "why has the process been so hard?" But I know well enough to know not question God's plan too much.

I would have to say graduate school was somewhat of a seamless process. The biggest challenge was my schedule. I was working 12-hour night shifts and in school during the day, I was literally flipping my sleep schedule every other day for a period of 2 years. Just as I neared the end of the program I had yet another major hurdle. I had to complete 500 clinical practice hours and was 100 away from the graduation requirement. Like I had done a few years before I went into panic mode and began to pool every resource I had. I spent day in and day out reaching out to strangers in the industry in hopes they would agree to allow me to precept with them for my final 100 hours. This process took more than 6 months. By now I had missed my original graduation date and was not able to walk the stage with my cohorts. In May of 2014 I secured a clinical practice location and completed the final piece of my graduate requirements.

August 2014, I walked the stage. I accomplished the goal of obtaining my Masters in nursing with a concentration in Family Nurse Practitioner and certification in Nursing Education. I was so proud and excited because I was one step closer to my dream of being able to take care of children just like "baby doctors." My dreams were coming true right before my eyes. It was amazing. I was able to appreciate it even greater because of the challenges I faced.

Prior to graduation, I applied for my first Nurse practitioner job and was hired immediately after interviewing. My mind was blown, I had no idea how it was going to be, but I had to jump in. All was going well, however I had not obtained my official license certification yet. I knew I had a good grasp on the information. I took a review course and studied leisurely while working full time as a brand new Nurse practitioner. I was learning a lot, getting to know the patients, families, and medical management style of the practice. The time came for me to sit for my licensure examination and guess what happened. I failed. I was literally devastated. Everything began to fall apart in my head. I was afraid to tell my boss and coworkers because I did not know if I was going to get fired, what would I do? I relocated to a new city, I had bills, and I had to support myself. What was I going to do? You know me, I kicked it into gear yet again. I began to study like crazy. I refused to let this be the end of my story, no way, no how. My job was amazing during this time and allowed me extra time off to study. About 30 days later, I sat for the examination again. This time, I passed. Thank the Lord, I had passed. I knew deep down that God would never set me up to fail but was continuously teaching me lessons. These lessons would afford me the testimony needed to help others who have hit a roadblock or two, or three. These lessons are the basis of my character, the have helped mold me into who I am.

About 5 years ago I began to feel the pull toward entrepreneurship. I believe I have always had the entrepreneurial spirit. As a young child when I decided I wanted to be a "baby doctor," I then also decided I wanted to own my own practice. I hadn't really though a lot about it after that moment. I went through all the motions of schooling, working, accomplishing goals, only for it to re-emerge in my spirit. God lit an itty-bitty fire for entrepreneurship in me; he also began to send people my way to confirm my assignment. Gaining clarity allowed me to understand my PURPOSE and the reason I was placed on this earth. That purpose is to touch others in such a positive way that they will never forget but will carry with them for the rest of their lives.

This brings about the real challenge, how in the world am I going to do that, how am I going to touch others in a positive manner? About two years ago that flame commenced to grow. I began to become uncomfortable in my secure place I had built. I was becoming unhappy with my daily routine; while patient care was rewarding, it just was not enough. I remember thinking to myself, "nursing isn't enough anymore, WHAT NOW?" That was a very hard pill to swallow and honestly to this day I am still dealing with it.

NOW WHAT

What now is the biggest and BEST part of my story. I am now in the middle of the what now and what next phase of my journey. The journey began with lots of personal development and self-discovery. Remember I spoke about perseverance, this is gong to be a huge part of any entrepreneurial journey. My first tip if you want to become an entrepreneur is to learn yourself. Do you have the ability to face challenges and keep going? Can you handle rejection? Learn what makes you tick and take time to just feel and be. The nursing profession can be very taxing, you constantly put your feelings aside to care for others. It is extremely important to pour back into yourself. You will hear me say over and over to remember your "Why". You must know why you are in this in order to do what is going to truly make you happy. Self-discovery is gaining insight into your own character. What makes me happy? Am I open-minded? Do I see myself as a success? If I had a billion dollars how would I spend it? All these self-discovery questions help you determine if you are satisfied with your life and can help guide you on the correct path.

Learning your triggers, good and bad, make it easy for you to decide if you are in the right place and or even the right career. Discovering your "Why" will save you lots of time and energy. I believe people go into nursing with good intentions but end up unhappy and frustrated, which shows daily during their interactions with patients and fellow coworkers. No one wants to be cared for by someone who they feel does not want to deal with them. Again, this is where knowing yourself will be very beneficial. Do you love answering questions and giving advice? Do you love educating? Do you love taking care of patients that are sedated or undergoing an operation? Do you like a fast paced, ever-changing environment? Get to know yourself and what you want out of your career.

Once you have discovered what your likes and dislikes are then you need to use those to begin to brainstorm. What is it that you want to do? Is it within nursing or outside of nursing. There is nothing wrong with wanting to do something outside of nursing. While nursing likely plays a huge part in your life that does not mean you must center your business around it. It is perfectly fine to find another business venture. Do you want just a side hustle or do you want to work for yourself full-time? I have met Nurses that are travel agents, success coaches, authors, jewelry or apparel designers, stylists, and the list goes on. So, the second step in what now is to decide what you want your business to be. For me, that does involve nursing in some aspect. I have become a serial entrepreneur, which means I have multiple business dealings. After deciding to step from behind the chart, the business ideas began to flow and that little fire I mentioned started growing even more!

    I prayed to God to lead me in the direction I should go. I was first led to write my first book. Couch to Career Becoming a Nurse was birthed out of the frustration with the process I went through when I decided to become a Nurse. It was a very natural decision because knowledge on all the steps that needed to be taken were not widely available. At the time, I was overwhelmed with all the options of school and the over-saturation of nursing information on the internet; therefore, I wanted the focus of Couch to Career to be on the steps to become a Nurse. I wanted to create a guide to ease the process, point people in the right direction, and give them clarity. A guide, blueprint, or strategy if you will, was the purpose behind Couch to Career Becoming a Nurse. The learning curve for writing and self- publishing a book is enormous, but I was up for the job because I knew I was doing it for a greater cause. It took lots of time and dedication to learn the steps I needed to follow to make the book happen. Shortly after writing, self-publishing, and becoming an Amazon New Releases Best Seller, my focus shifted.

DESTINED FOR GREATNESS

My next goal was to develop a network where Nurses and student Nurses could come together outside of the hospital and be able to develop themselves in their career life and personal life. Savvi Society Ltd. is just that. Within Savvi Society I am known as the Chief Savvi Officer and I function as a Health Careers Consultant. I use my knowledge and expertise to help aspiring healthcare professionals get into the program of their desires or attain the job of their dreams. Within Savvy Society, I offer consulting and coaching services for those who desire personalized assistance. The network is available for anyone likes to learn and grow at their own pace and just need the tools to help take them to the next level. My mission, as stated before, is to positively impact the lives of so many people that I will no longer be able to count. I also desire to improve every life that I touch! That being said, my next tip for those who want to become a Nurse entrepreneur is to have a clear purpose behind starting your business. Is the purpose of your business to serve others, or are you doing it for selfish reasons? Think long and hard about it.

Now will you allow me to share a secret with you? It was not until a few years ago I began to act on the pull towards entrepreneurship. It sat on the back burner while God continued to groom me for this. This venture would completely take me out of my comfort zone. Nursing comes easy to me, teaching comes easy to me, coaching and motivating comes easy to me, but opening a physical "brick and mortar" business does not come so easy. I incorporated True Calling Healthcare & Training back in 2015. I allowed it to lie dormant for the last few years, but True Calling is now my most recent focus. True Calling Healthcare & Training is a home care agency with a training division. This training division houses the Certified Nurse Assistant School, a compassionate training program for healthcare professionals which also offers community trainings for caregivers to help be best equipped to care for their loved ones. My purpose behind this business is to help build up the foundation of nursing, i.e. Nursing Assistants, and to provide top-notch quality care for those who need it at home.

This business is particularly very near and dear to me as it is a part of a family that kept my grandparents' home until end of life. My grandparents were very independent their entire 90+ years on this planet. It was not until my grandfather passed that my grandmother needed us to all pitch in to care for her. I had relocated about two hours from them but was there almost every week to help. I knew what it was like to care for people at the end of life, but was experiencing being on the other end of that for the first time. I really got to see firsthand how hard it was to balance work and caring for a loved one both full-time.

Do you see the pattern yet? If you see a void, fill it. That is my next tip for becoming a Nurse entrepreneur. Finding voids that you can fill is the best way to transition into the next phase of your career. Every business I have started, I've done so because it was something I wish I had at some point throughout my life. I wish I had a road map, so I created one. I wish I had a network within nursing, so I created one. I wish I had someone I could trust to care for my loved ones so, I created a company that does that as well. I have chosen to do so while continuing to working the field. I am sure you will see throughout this book you do not have to leave nursing to become a Nursepreneur as I like to call us. You can continue working and still run a business if you desire. There are no rules and the possibilities are endless! This leads me to my next tip. Execution. Execution is key.

EXECUTION

The third tip in the process is execution. To properly execute, you must develop a team. I talk a lot about team building these days because it is uber important in so many areas of your life. There is no one who can go through this entrepreneurial journey alone; you need a team. No rules necessarily apply for who should be on your team, but my suggestion would be to know your strengths and weaknesses and build your team around those. Are you very organized but lack creativity? Are you good with numbers but writing isn't your strong suit? Do ideas come easily to you but the steps to execute do not? Your team should be able to compliment you and help pull your vision together.

You, my future Nurseprenuer will also need team members that are there solely for support purposes. You will need someone who can pray with you when you need it, encourage you to keep going when you want to quit, and bounce ideas off and they tell you, nope, that's terrible. Team members would be honest, trust worthy, and hard working; or at least that is what I look for in a team. I personally don't want "yes men" on my team. I need someone to tell me those colors are ugly and do not work well together. I am not saying my team is perfect, but they are very good because we have been able to accomplish a lot in s short amount of time.

The second tip that goes along with execution is research. Research may be the most important part of this entire process. Are you reinventing the wheel or just perfecting a spoke? Once you have your business idea you need to know what else is going on in the world that could be like your idea. If you happen to not find anything and you are a pioneer in your business then kudos to you! You then get to invent the wheel. Again, there are no rights or wrongs, you just need to know what is out there and if it seems to have/be working. You cannot start anything without doing research; if that is not your strong suit, then guess what? Have a team member who can get it done! However, I find it very hard to believe that you are not a good researcher. A large part of nursing is research and investigation. If you can do it for your patients, you can do it for your business.

Naturally the next step in execution is developing the plan to execute. This requires you to thoroughly think through the "how" of your business. You should begin to map out the steps to get you from where you are to where you want to be. This is where you begin to develop the strategy behind your business and is an invaluable step. Being transparent, this is the step I had to revisit and I feel is the reason so many businesses fail. It is not that their business is not great; it may simply be that they lacked strategy and were not able to execute effectively. In this short chapter; I will not be able to do you justice on creating a strategy, but I will say this. Invest your time in the strategy behind your business, please.

Moving forward, the final part of execution is follow-through. You need discipline to be able to follow through with what needs to be done. What good is having a business idea and developing a team if there is no follow-through? Follow-through is the key to getting you from step A to step B. Nothing will ever get done if you are a starter and never a finisher. Being able to complete tasks no matter how you feel is what being an entrepreneur is all about. You need that discipline to kick in when your motivation is wearing off. You can't ever let your discipline fade if you are going to make it as an entrepreneur. So, if you lack in that area, it's time to get it whipped into shape. Remember that your results are based on your effort.

My final tip for those who want to become an entrepreneur is to rely on your faith and spirituality. Get in touch with your spiritual side if you haven't already because you will need it. You are going to be doing things that you have never imagined you would be able to. I make sure to pray over my businesses every day. I pray about literally every step. Who should I work with, who should I hire, where will my clients come from? Everything. I pray about what my next steps should and will be, and even who is coming with me on the journey. In addition to prayer, you need to practice gratitude. Gratitude is the quality of feeling or being grateful or thankful. I don't know about you but, I am grateful for everything I get my hands on. I try to be the best steward I can so that I am consistently blessed with more. Also remember to keep those around that can offer you spiritual support as well. I am sure to reach out in times of trials and ask for my support system to agree with me in prayer. Sometimes I don't even ask but they just send me a message that keeps me inspired and motivated.

One last bonus tip is networking. Network, network, network, then network some more. Networking helps to build your support system. Networking is now more easily accessible because we are in the age of social media and you can become acquaintances with anyone across the world. Get out and meet other entrepreneurs. Go out and meet other Nurseprenuers as well. That has been one of the best things I could have ever started. I made a vow to myself that I would broaden my horizon and start meeting new people; not to mention, I relocated to a city where I only knew my significant other. Thus, my mission network began. I have since made several new friends and connections via social media that led to me meeting people in person that live in my area. I have met a network of fellow Nurses in my city, home care owners in and out of my area, and other current and aspiring entrepreneurs, as well as Nursepreneurs. I have even gain mentors through networking. This support system I have built has been able to offer words of advice and encouragement. This has afforded me the ability to literally have any question answered, create a solution for any problem I have, and get feedback on the things that I am working on. Networking has been the paramount of my business success thus far. You too should build a network of people who have been and are going where you want to go.

MOVING FORWARD

If you are reading this and you're a Nurse interested in becoming an entrepreneur, no matter if it is full or part time, all you need to remember is this - never let anyone place you in a box. I am sure everyone in this book can agree on what I am about to say. At some point through the journey, someone will ask you, "Nurses make good money, why would you want to start a business?" To me, what they are saying is be comfortable where you are, ignore that urge to do more, shut up, and be happy with your job. Not everyone will understand your choice, not everyone will support it. Your closest friends or family may not even understand. Do not let that stop you. Your dream is your dream for a reason. It is not for anyone else to "get." Never settle for something just because society says it is how things should be.

When you face challenges (and you will), think back about my story, think about how there were challenges that could have taken me completely off course. Let that inspire you to stick with it and never give up. Things do not often come easily, and that is okay, that does not mean you should not have it, it just means you will have to work for it. If this is something you are passionate about, let our stories and words of encouragement motivate you to move forward and pursue your dreams. I am a firm believer if you can be a Nurse, you can be anything you set your mind to. We create our own realities, we make are own rules. I was not produced from a cookie cutter and neither were you. Good luck as you begin the journey into entrepreneurship!

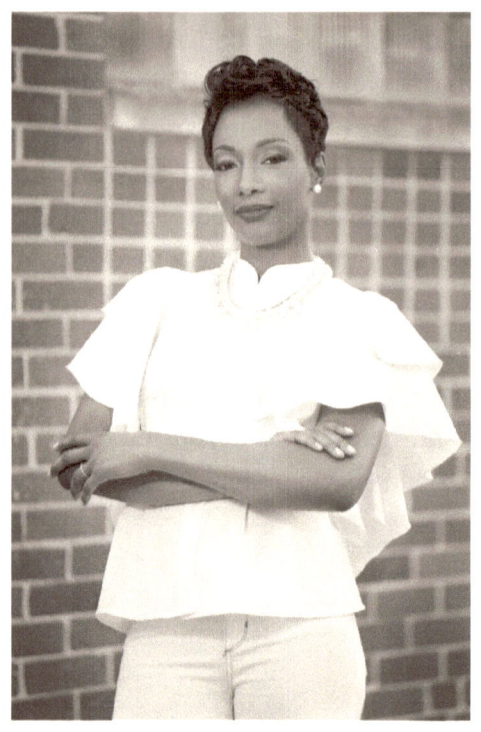

About The Author

Jeteia prides herself on being someone who had a clear vision for her future since the age of 5. She always knew she wanted to serve others in the medical field. Knowing her career direction early on blessed her with the ability to achieve her first major career goal at the age of 26, becoming a Nurse.

Upon reaching this accomplishment, she quickly began serving in the pediatric ICU step-down unit at 2 of the top 10 hospitals in the United States. In 2014, she would reach her next career goal of becoming a Nurse Practitioner. Jeteia has always had a love for educating and decided that her way of giving back to the profession would be serving as a nursing instructor, while continuing to practice medicine. Though she enjoyed her work, she felt that for the first time that she had hit a career glass ceiling and wasn't so clear on her next move.

She knew she wanted to continue to serve, but there was a burning passion that told her, this time she needed to take that passion a step further. To be effective in a way that helped others excel in reaching their aspirations and be in good health requires some creativity. Through this process Savvi Society was created. The content for Savvi Society was created specifically for those interested in healthcare but need a bit of guidance, motivation, and support. Jeteia was also able to turn her passion for home health into a business by opening True Calling Healthcare & Training a home care based agency in the local community. True Calling Healthcare & Training will also serve as a certified nursing assistant training facility and a community educational facility for those who need to learn more about caring for their loved ones at home. Jeteia is determined to impact the world through Savvi Society and True Calling Healthcare & Training.

For more information:

Follow the Savvi movement on Instagram/Twitter @jeteiab

Facebook @ Savvi Society, Ltd.

Follow True Calling Healthcare & Training, LLC on Instagram and Facebook @truecallinghealth

TRUSTING MY JOURNEY:
Inspirational stories of Nurse Entrepreneurs

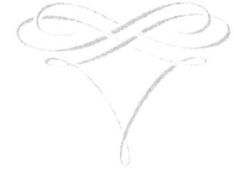

BY
BRITTANY WINESTOCK APRN, FNP-BC

INTRODUCTION

Nursing is a calling, a passion, a gift, a service. Nursing is so many things. A Nurse to me is caring, compassionate, an advocate for the patient and family; knowledgeable, and so much more.

As a young girl, I always knew I wanted to do something to impact others; something in the healthcare field. It was not until my mother became ill, that I realized nursing was the path for me. I went to many appointments, and hospital stays with my mother. During those times, she would always express how she felt as though the physicians were in and out of her room so quickly. She felt as though she was not being heard. She would question, "how can I properly receive treatment, when no one has the time to listen to my concerns?" She then experienced a caring group of Nurses who listened to her concerns. I remember the difference in how my mother felt and responded; based on the level of care she received. She spoke very highly of the Nurses she encountered. I was overwhelmed with the amount of compassion those Nurses showed, and I wanted to be that for someone and their family. After research, I decided I wanted to be a Nurse Practitioner as this would allow me to provide care and compassion, while having the ability to prescribe and treat.

After graduating high school I went straight to nursing school that fall and began this amazing journey in my life. As you may know, there is not anything easy about nursing school. I recall feeling defeated; considering I was used to easily excelling from kindergarten throughout twelfth grade. I had just turned 18 years old and was learning so much about myself. I was living on my own for the first time; and attending a school with other top students; it was just…. Different!!! The nursing school I attended required completion of pre-requisites and was based on your GPA; the top 32 students were selected to enter the nursing program the upcoming school year. I remember clearly missing out on college events with my friends as I sat in my dorm room studying for hours. Late nights and early mornings was my new routine. This is not how I imagined college. I knew that it would not be easy, but I thought that I would be able to enjoy myself.

As becoming a Nurse was my goal, I strived hard to gain the highest GPA in my prerequisite courses with hopes of being accepted into the upcoming nursing school year. I took Chemistry 101 and 102, Biology 101 and 102, Anatomy and Physiology, and a few other standard courses. I remember many tears that first year; and spending many days outside of my Chemistry and Biology professors' office. I will never forget studying hours for my first Chemistry exam, to receive a grade of a "D". I was horrified. A "D" I can't make a "D". This is what led to many discussions with my professor to gain a better understanding of this subject. It eventually paid off and I completed the course with a B +. Hard work truly pays off. My freshman year was an adjustment, but I made it!!!!

That summer I was excited to be home with family and friends; but I could not relax as I was stressfully waiting on the letter from the school of nursing. Well, that summer day came and I could not even open the letter myself. I remember sitting on my parent's bed with my mother, as my father read what it said. We would like to congratulate and welcome you into the school of nursing at Lander University. I cried, as my hard work had paid off!!!!

Entering the nursing program was pure excitement and then the work came. We had class Monday, Wednesday, Friday, and clinical every Tuesday and Thursday that required medication cards on all patients, preplanning we called it; and care plans after each clinical. This was along with all of our other courses, test, homework assignments, etc. I thought to myself, "what have I gotten myself into?" I knew that I needed a strict and very detailed plan to succeed with this level of requirements. Oh, the many days of trial and error of studying, note cards, drawing pictures, creating songs, and any other ways to hopefully retain and understand all the provided information. I would question to myself, "is it even humanly possible to learn and know this amount of information???" For those of you wondering, it is possible. It requires hard work, dedication, and a plan.

Fast forwarding through undergraduate school and the NCLEX. I have successfully overcome those hurdles and it is time to begin working as a Nurse. I started in a hospital that I loved as it was faith based, on a medical-surgical unit working twelve hour shifts, 3 days a week. WOW, what an amazing schedule I was twenty-one years old and able to care for people just as I wanted. This unit provided me with the foundation that I knew I needed, and ultimately molded me into the Nurse I am today. I worked on this unit for a couple of years and then started working in the PRN float pool. Now, that I had a strong foundation I wanted to expand my knowledge. I am always striving to grow and learn. I began working on every telemetry unit in our hospital (I worked for a cardiac hospital). I gained so much from this. I loved the flexible schedule and the choice of which unit I was going to work; all while gaining more knowledge. During this time, I had my first daughter, got married, and started graduate school to continue working on my goal of becoming a Nurse practitioner.

Throughout both undergrad and graduate school, I was always a great student. It didn't come easy by any means, but I worked hard and performed well. Graduate school was a bit different as I was now a wife, mother, full-time Nurse, and full-time student. I had to revise my schedule to incorporate all these things in my life. I needed every minute.

I would get up early every morning to study and complete homework, SOAP notes, and any other assignments before it was time to wake my kids to prepare for the day. I would then get them ready and go to work. After getting home and getting them to bed for the night; I would spend more time studying, completing homework, and finishing assignments. While maintaining all those roles, I remained consistent and did well.

Then test-taking time would come around and I would become extremely anxious and overwhelmed. This was one of my greatest hurdles during this process. I wanted to succeed so much that each test was stressful. One vivid memory is the board-certifying exam for the NCLEX, but mostly the Family Nurse Practitioner certification. I followed all the standard testing tips; get a good night of sleep, eat a good breakfast, know your route to the testing center… I did all the above. I walked into the testing center with my required material and instantly felt my stomach churning. The anxiety started. When you walk in the desk clerk requests your information and allows you to put your personal belongings in a locker. Next, you are instructed to take a seat and wait to be called. As, the proctor called my name, I thought I would pass out. This is the part that really sent me over the edge. I had to stand in this box outlined with tape. I was then instructed to stick my hands in my pockets and pull them out to show that I did not have any materials in my pockets. I was then asked to pull up the leg of my pants, so that she could assess my ankles for any material. Lastly, the metal detector… At this point, I was sick. As you are seated in the testing center, you receive a few more rules. All that I wanted to do at that point was to get the test over with.

It was finally time for me to test. Many thoughts flooded my mind, JNC-7, Asthma stepwise approach, diabetes, lab values, it was all running together. I took a deep breath and prayed. Each question I could feel the anxiety increasing. I felt as though I did not know anything. Oh, I have seen that before; but I don't remember. Oh, wait let me go back to question number five. So many things went through my mind, other than focusing. This eventually led to me failing my Family Nurse Practitioner (FNP) board certification. With the FNP certification exam, it is different from the NCLEX as you receive your results the same day. I walked out of the testing center and signed out; as the proctor printed my results. She notarized the paper for what seemed to be hours. When she handed me the paper; I glanced down and read, "We regret to inform you…" I failed. I failed by 5 points. 5, yes 5 points!!!! I was absolutely broken. I remember sitting in my SUV in the parking lot of the testing center, crying my eyes out.

I could not believe that this was happening to me. I could not understand why I was having such difficulty when I knew the information. I had spent numerous hours studying, reviewing, missing out on family activities, and the list goes on. What did I do wrong? There is no way I can pass if I spent all that time studying and failed. What more does it take to pass? I spent many days beating myself up and trying to figure out how I was going to move forward. What would people think? How could I disappoint my family? Will I pass the next time? You know… all the crazy thoughts that we go through during times like these.

I then decided, enough was enough and I began to figure out how I would succeed; failure was NOT an option. I was always one to come up with a song, mnemonic, joke, or any tactic to retain the nursing material. As you know, there is TONS of information that must be learned to become a Nurse/Nurse Practitioner, so I worked to make it fun and easier for myself. I realized that if I knew the material backward and forwards, then even under pressure (test anxiety) I would still succeed.

To catch you up a bit, during graduate school I began working in case management developing programs for the same hospital so that I could work Monday through Fridays. This was a better schedule for family, school, and work to balance. After graduating I began to teach now that I had a Master of Science in Nursing. I taught BSN and FNP students (online, in the classroom, and clinically). I did this while working to pass my certification exam.

This became the turning point for me. I found myself utilizing the same tactics that I used for myself with my students. I would teach them how to study, and review in an easier manner. I lived by the importance of KNOWING the information and not just memorizing it. I also found myself giving them advice on how to work the hours they had in a day to study, complete school work, work full-time or part-time jobs, and be involved with family.

I soon found out it was working for my students as well. My students would often say, "Mrs. Winestock, you make this so easy. You should do review courses." I heard them, but I continued with my day-to-day norms. I was so busy working, studying, and being a wife and mother that I truly was not listening to what they were showing me. They were showing me that my tactics worked!!! Finally, I decided to test again and successfully passed; I then realized maybe my tactics do work. Maybe these students are on to something.

Well, I am a firm believer in everything happening for a reason and that God guides our paths. Those that know me also know that my mottos are "Trust the journey" and Philippians 4:13 which states, "I can do all things through Christ who strengthens me." So, when I look back over my life; this is all a part of my journey that has brought me to the point of Nurse entrepreneurship. I went through school; I worked as a nursing assistant; I took boards; I failed boards; while waiting to retake boards I taught students; and all of this provided me with the foundation needed to create The Nursing Studio.

During the time of hardship, I could not understand why everything I faced was so difficult. I couldn't see what the outcome would be. The one thing I did was continued to work hard and to believe that it would all work in my favor. Now, each step displays where I am today. Things aren't easy in this phase either, but it is all building blocks to the next level.

WHY I CHOSE NURSE ENTREPRENEURSHIP…

As we grow and mature in life, our personal desires change. Originally, working three twelve- hour shifts was perfect for me; then, I had a husband and children and that option was no longer the best for my family and me. I needed more time in the evenings; so I could pick up my daughters from school/daycare, and do homework, cook dinner, give baths, etc. I switched to a Monday through Friday 8-hour a day job. This worked for my family, but I still wanted more for myself, career wise. Also, as some of you may find relative to your own lives, Monday through Friday isn't the most convenient schedule either. With small children, it is difficult to alter your schedule for frequent appointments; it requires you to take off from work. I just needed something to balance it all for me. Well, don't we all!

I wanted a job where I could still be involved with both patients and students, but also spend as much time as possible with my family. Where do you find something like this??? You don't; you create it! So, what I decided to do was work clinically and become a Nurse entrepreneur also.

I chose to become a Nurse entrepreneur because I felt as though other Nurses/Nurse practitioners, aspiring Nurses, and Nursing students needed the same guidance I needed while on that journey. I wanted to provide them with what I had wished was provided to me. What better way to make this happen, than to simply do it!!!

I started out gradually by mentoring students, Nurses, and Nurse practitioners. I also provided career specific resumes, career tips, job and salary negotiation, and most of all tactics to easily retain the nursing material they needed.

As, I continued to work with reviewers, more and more people began to reach out to me. To my surprise, people really wanted my services and appreciated what I had to offer. To this day, I still get chills when working with each reviewer. I love to see it "click" for them; what once was difficult, suddenly becomes simple. I love receiving those messages that say, "Thank you Brittany, I passed!" These very things made me realize I was doing exactly what I needed to be doing at that very time. Trust the journey!

Have you realized that as a Nurse, you can tell anyone about your day or your experience, and they do not truly understand? Only a Nurse can comprehend the magnitude of another Nurse's day or experience. I wanted to provide that support to another person following this journey. There is nothing better than having someone that relates to you.

While on my journey of becoming a Nurse and Nurse practitioner, I dreamed of something or someone to guide me. My instructors were amazing, but outside of the classroom I needed more. I wanted a way to organize, review, and retain the large amounts of information provided. I did not want to skip over information or memorize information just to get through the test. I wanted to KNOW the material so that I could effectively implement all my knowledge, to impact and save others' lives.

To do this, I needed a condensed yet thorough system. I also would run into days when I wished I could reach out to someone for guidance. I craved someone with true compassion who could provide honest direction throughout my nursing career. I ran into a few ladies who not only became mentors, but friends. I wanted something that offered this for all Nurses and aspiring Nurses. I wanted a way to make a community to no longer "eat our young", but to uplift, guide, and support one another. The only way for this to happen in this exact manner was to create this opportunity!!

Nursing entrepreneurship allows me to offer exactly what I want and need in a manner, which upholds my values; in hopes of impacting others and advancing the career of nursing overall.

Nurse entrepreneurship allows me the gratification that I desired. I not only get to work clinically at a hospital while providing patient care, but I also impact nursing. I am blessed with the chance to assist students and mentor them into and throughout nursing school. I get to see people who were discouraged and failing major exams transform into appreciative students/reviewers who are passing examinations. Receiving testimonials alone is gratification to me. When I receive a referral, the feeling is priceless. My hard work and struggles are paying off by supporting someone else along their journey.

To top all of this off as a wife and mother of two (with one on the way), flexibility is a major need. As you may be able to relate; I wanted to create a way to do what I love, while not missing out on what matters most to me… my family!!! Entrepreneurship allows for flexibility while still doing what you love. Also, I strive to be a great example for my children. I want them to always know that you can do anything you set your mind and hard work always pays off. That is why I chose Nurse entrepreneurship.

THE NURSING STUDIO

I, Brittany Winestock, am the founder and CEO of The Nursing Studio. I am a test-taking tactician. I provide students, graduates, anxious testers, testers who have previously failed, and reviewers with tactics to easily retain and successfully pass examinations.

The Nursing Studio is not only a place to review and study, but also a community for like-minded Nurses, Nurse practitioners, Nursing students, and aspiring Nurses to support one another on their nursing journey.

The Nursing Studio offers many resources, courses, activities, and packages to support your every need. There are courses for Nurses and Nurse practitioners to prepare for certifying board examinations. There are also courses to aid students through nursing or NP school. The Nursing Studio currently has a 97% pass rate for the NCLEX and 100% pass rate for the FNP board (AANP and ANCC).

The beauty of The Nursing Studio is that you have the option for one-on-one review sessions where you are assisted based on your needs rather than standardization. The Nursing Studio offers many ways to engage and get involved with your nursing community. We offer two groups on Facebook, where one is geared for Nurses, Nursing students, and aspiring Nurses and the other is for Nurse Practitioners preparing for boards. You can find these groups listed on Facebook as The Nursing Studio and The Nursing Studio: Nurse Practitioner Board Survival Group. We have one community on Instagram @TheNursingStudio and you can find everything you need on our website: www.thenursingstudio.org.

Although this business has been successful; I do not want it to seem as though entrepreneurship comes easy. There will be roadblocks; life will happen, but remain consistent and strive for your goals.

On my business journey, it is definitely hard work as now I am balancing working for a hospital and simultaneously running my own business. I find myself using the schedule from studying for my business. I work early mornings and late nights after my family is asleep to create content, design courses, review and research material, and the list goes on. I do all these things so that I can enhance my business; with the hopes of eventually cutting back on my work hours. Now when I launch courses, conduct workshops, post motivation and test taking tips, it seems like the picture-perfect role. There is backend work that is required for those outcomes.

I say all this to say that you will still work hard. We all work hard in different ways. As the saying goes, "It will never seem like work, when you are doing your passion." So, it is hard work, but a different kind of hard work. It is enjoyable, gratifying, inspiring, and so much more.

Do not allow the work to distract you because the outcome will come. Use those as stepping-stones to eventually see the fruits of your labor. Also, know that when you look to your role model, it may seem that they have it all together and some days they do; but it took work, hurdles, mistakes, obstacles, and successes to reach that outcome. My thought process is if you do it right the first time and give it your all; you will never have to do that again. You will have to tweak things to remain relevant; but you will not have to put in that same amount of time and effort.

TIPS FOR ASPIRING NURSE ENTREPRENEURS OR ANY ENTREPRENEUR

As with anything else, entrepreneurship is far from easy. It takes lots of hard work, time, and dedication. You are a Nurse, so I know you know all about that. Entrepreneurship is currently on the rise in our society. I think you must first separate the thought of financial gain and work for your passion. To CONSISTENTLY provide hard work and dedication, there must be some type of passion to fuel you.

I am often asked how I decided the correct path to take on my entrepreneurial journey. I always advise Nurse entrepreneurs or aspiring Nurse entrepreneurs to find what you are truly passionate about and your gifts. Do not start a business to simply have a business. Do what drives you. This is what will make your journey enjoyable and worth the work.

Next, how will the business impact others and what is your market? Go through each step, research, and have a true understanding of how you want to start. Everything does not need to be perfect to start, but you do need direction. Entrepreneurship requires strategies, plans, and consistency to remain on course. The beauty is that everything that you do in your business; will be a personal accomplishment. You will see the fruits of your labor.

Here are eight tips to hopefully guide you on your entrepreneurial journey!

1. Focus on your Passion. Chose something that you are passionate about and involves your personal gifts. Strive to become an expert in that area. This allows you to put a dollar to your service and actually have people who benefit from your service.

2. Always do your best. Life is busy, nursing is busy, and entrepreneurship is busy. Although your roles can be time consuming, you must provide your best at all times. This is YOUR business and YOUR brand, so you want ALL your work to speak for your true abilities.

3. Time management: Again, life is busy, nursing is busy, and entrepreneurship is busy. So, you must adequately plan your time. Time is very valuable, and should not be wasted. Set specific goals and deadlines and stick with it. This will allow you to be most effective in your business and maintain balance in your life.

4. Consistency: Consistency is key in anything. Someone who is consistent can conquer anything. It may not happen immediately and you may become discouraged; but if you will remain consistent, you will see the fruits of your labor.

5. Never forget why. Never forget why you decided to start this business. This will keep you engaged, passionate, humble, and most effective. When you forget your "why" your flame begins to dull; your fuel begins to run out.

6. Do NOT Compare. Do NOT compare yourself to anyone else. Everyone has different goals, progressions, achievements, etc. If you focus on what may seem to be better for someone else, then; you may miss your "better."

7. Trust the journey. Most of all, ALWAYS trust the journey. Your journey is exactly what is designed for you. Trust that. Enjoy each day and each milestone. Enjoy every accomplishment, no matter the size.

8. Never give up! If you are passionate and have a dream, never give up on that dream. No matter the obstacles you may reach, keep pushing!!!

I hope that my story and journey can be an inspiration to you and your journey! Take these tips and take one day at a time. Remember to trust the journey; there is a lesson in everything, and you have something to offer to any experience. I wish you much success in your Nurse entrepreneurial journey!

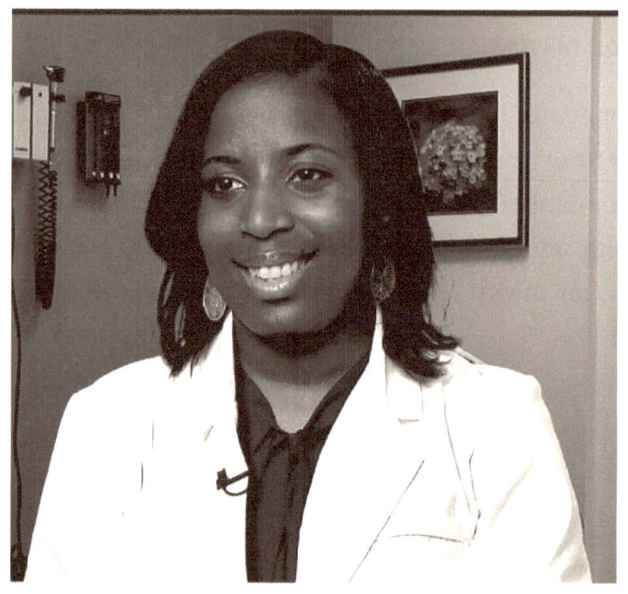

About the Author

Brittany Winestock is a Family Nurse Practitioner and Nurse entrepreneur. She has worked in healthcare for more than ten years. She is the founder and CEO of The Nursing Studio, where she is known as a test-taking tactician. She received this title as Brittany provides students, graduates, anxious testers, and reviewers with tactics to easily retain and successfully pass examinations. She also converts reviewers who previously failed an examination to passing that very same examination.

Brittany has a nursing background in medical-surgical nursing, cardiology, transitional care, and case management; her Nurse Practitioner background is family and works in cardiology. Brittany has started three successful programs; and serves as a guest speaker for university, church, and facility engagements. Brittany also teaches Nurses in the Bachelor of Science program, and Family Nurse Practitioners. She has taught in the clinical setting, online courses, and in the classrooms at the University of South Carolina, South University, and Grand Canyon University.

Brittany has many exciting upcoming events and courses in her career! Be on the lookout at what The Nursing Studio has coming!!!

FOR MORE INFORMATION CONTACT THE AUTHOR AT:

admin@thenursingstudio.org

FB: The Nursing Studio: The Nurse Practitioner Board Survival Group

IG: @thenursingstudio

Website: www.thenursingstudio.org

FROM SCRUBS TO PUMPS

BY
Melanie McCrary-Fuller BSN, RN

INTRODUCTION

Ten years ago, I was a Nurse with a handwritten dream, working the night shift with a cup of coffee and a plan; that would take six years to transfer from paper to reality.

Starting my healthcare care career as a Certified Nursing Assistant at the age of twenty-one after attending a four-week course was a quick way to contribute to my family. Becoming a certified nursing assistant would prove to play a life changing role in my life. I would go on to work as a Nursing Assistant for seven years. While employed at a local hospital during that time, I met several Nurses that motivated me to further my career; ultimately, I enrolled in a Practical Nursing Program and worked as an LPN for three years before registering in Charity School of Nursing LPN to RN program. This program began the first week of August 2005; and after only attending for three weeks, Hurricane Katrina hit New Orleans and changed the lives of those whom resided in our city forever. I evacuated to Atlanta, Georgia and secured a job as an LPN. Enthused by Atlanta's culture and room for growth, I decided that I wanted to purchase home there after completing school but, after five months, I was notified by a Charity School of Nursing instructor that class would resume. Determined to complete the program, I returned to New Orleans, and eight months later graduated as a Registered Nurse.

During my early years as a Registered Nurse, I worked on a Neuro Unit. Eager and fast to learn, I quickly became a leader on the unit; but advancement opportunities were scarce. New Nurses would enter my unit and transfer to specialty areas to become supervisors in less than a year of employment. My Nursing skills were perfected so I couldn't understand at the time why I wasn't I offered those promotions. The thing is it was not for me to understand at this stage of my life. I knew very early on that I had so much more to offer to the world of healthcare. My Nursing game was so tight and my skills were so proficient that I could run a code and save a life without sweating; but I was still working this twelve-hour shift. Co-workers told me that I was such a calm and calculated Nurse and would make a great Nursing Educator as I was often chosen to precept new Nurses, instead of Nurses employed much longer. But twelve-hour shifts were growing old and after the birth of my last child, I knew it was time to move on.

I came across a job posting for a Hospice Nurse and thought to myself, I could do that job. But hospice was such a depressing area of Nursing; how could I provide care to terminally ill patients daily? I was skeptical to accept a new job offer, I was working and had been in that position for almost 8 years. I learned in Nursing school the goal was to save lives. After contemplating for a few days, I finally interviewed for the job and was offered a full-time position. The next day I submitted a two-week notice and embarked upon a new career as a Hospice Registered Nurse Case Manager. I was excited to enter a new realm of Nursing that would offer quality end of life care. After seven years of working in the hospital, I left with a 401K check in the bank, a new Nursing role, and my handwritten plan still lingering in the back of my mind. During this time in my career, there were not many small private-owned Nursing schools in the New Orleans area. Of those schools, only two were owned by Nurses. I was too scared to contact any of the business owners for support or advice, so I turned to the internet as a guide. I began to research the schools whenever I had spare time, admiring those Nurses turned business owners. I would repeat daily, if they could do it successfully, I could too. I was consumed with the thought of being a boss, intertwined with the hope of leaving a legacy for my kids.

As a Hospice Nurse, I began to encounter many professional Nurses with advance degrees who held managerial positions. I was determined to learn as much as I could from these professional Nurses. Exerting management skills daily was a part of my job as a Hospice Case Manager; after three years as a Case Manager, I was offered a Director of Nursing position. But something was missing. I was helping other business owners live their dream, make their visions a reality, and breathing success into someone else's business while my own handwritten plan was tucked away in my pocket. Every day I thought to myself, I will execute my plan in two months, then two months would become four months. The time was now; it was time for me to birth my vision and live my dream. But how would I start the business? I had no idea where to turn. I again turned to the internet to Google as much information as possible.

I researched the guidelines and regulations for my city and state as it related to the business I was starting. I was told the first thing I would need to get started was a physical location. Purchasing a building was not a profitable option, so I chose to lease. I began to search for a building by starting small and found something within my budget. I could negotiate the first few months of rent in exchange for my husband to make the necessary repairs and freshly paint the unit. The next step was choosing a name for the school. This step was probably the hardest; I spent so much time trying to decide on a name. I initially chose West Bank Professional Nursing Training, but after more research, I discovered that it was too lengthy to brand; and because West Bank is a parish within the city, multiple businesses started with the title West Bank. I also learned that if possible, start your business title with the letter A so your business would always be listed at the top of any directory. With the help of a friend who gave me the name Advanced, from which I would ultimately decide to drop the ED, the school name was formed Advance Nursing Training. I opted for Nursing because my goal is to stick to Nursing and only offer Nursing courses for Certified Nursing Assistant and Practical Nursing.

As a state regulation to start a proprietary school, I had to formulate a business plan. I had no idea how I was going to write a business plan, but with the help of my husband and Google, I prepared a business plan. I did not want to take out any loans so I continued to work every day. With my retirement from the hospital in savings and the financial help of my husband and his parents, my dream began to unfold. While working every day from eight to five, I would go home in the evening and dedicate time to establishing my business. The requirements were lengthy and exhausting. I would go to bed after midnight for days at a time, sparking arguments between my spouse and me. Someone told me once, you will work harder for your business vs. working for someone else. I was learning very early that the quotes were true. Every job I held taught me a lesson about entrepreneurship - the encounter with a physician, the handling of a family complaint, and the gift of the importance of teamwork amongst fellow co-workers. I knew I wasn't born a businesswoman; but by observation, trial and error, and hard work, I was becoming one. I did not become a Nurse Entrepreneur by chance; I became a Nurse Entrepreneur because of a gift - the gift of acquired knowledge, the gift to learn, the gift to teach, and the gift to inspire. All are gifts from God.

It was important for me to follow my dream and share the journey with others. I was inspired by so many Nurses along the way and felt it was my turn to give upcoming Nurses someone to look to and say if she can do it, then I can too. After many tears, doors being closed, and late nights in bed writing business plans with my husband, I did it. My school, Advance Nursing Training, opened in 2013 as a proprietary school serving individuals interested in becoming Certified Nursing Assistants. My first class consisted of only five students. I treated those five students as if I had a class of fifty. Committed to instilling the importance of professionalism and compassion, those five students were compelled to continue their careers after Advance Nursing Training.

Shortly after my first class I connected with the local workforce agency in my area. The agency is structured to assist unemployed individuals with job training to successfully gain employment. I registered my school and met all requirements to participate in this program. I received maybe a total of ten students in a one-year span. I later learned that students were deterred away from certain schools and coerced to attend other schools. I was hurt to learn that agencies would promote such a disservice to the school and unfairness to the students who should have a choice to choose their qualified school of choice. When brought to the agency's attention, I learned that Certified Nursing Assistant schools would be removed from the list due to not meeting the state's list as a top demand occupation. I am not aware of another occupation you can train for in three weeks and gain employment in less than forty- five days, but the workforce program came to an end.

    Left with doubt of how we would fill our class with only private pay students, I began to network and market the school through social media, friends, attending community outreach event, and churches. The school enrollment never decreased; but I knew if that door closed, then another would open. While having a conversation with a close friend, I learned that a community nonprofit organization was establishing a parent educator program in addition to the daycare program they were already offering. My friend suggested I meet with someone she knew who was assisting with the program and present the idea that my school would make a great collaboration opportunity. I set up a meeting and introduced the school's curriculum. I later received a call that the partnership was approved. Every event and encounter has a reason and will occur at a given season. The students I met through this partnership became my motivation and inspiration to continue to pursue my dreams. My staff and I have become parents at times as well as mentors, probation officers, counselors and babysitters. We have had over two hundred students complete our program and successfully gain employment as Certified Nursing Assistants. After a year, I was notified that the nonprofit organization no longer had funding for the partnership. This time I was not bothered with how we would fill our classroom seats; by now I had a clear understanding that I was not in control. If a door closes, lock it; I knew I would receive a key to open another door.

I no longer stress about enrollment; the school's reputation speaks for itself. Former students of the school became our biggest marketing tool. At Advance Nursing Training, the staff and myself continue to multi-task as instructors, moms, motivators, and professional role models to our students. We are here for that student seeking guidance academically and emotionally. Deeply connected and committed to the community, Advance Nursing continues to partner with several programs to assist young moms in the New Orleans area. As I move forward into the school's fourth anniversary, I have continued to pursue my dream of starting a Practical Nursing program, which was my sole purpose of opening the school. Having contemplated closing the school many times in the last two years, I am thankful to have positive people in my circle, encouraging me to continue and cheering me along the way. I recently began the accreditation procedure, a costly and lengthy process, which is a state requirement prior to starting a Practical Nursing program.

The task of establishing a business and becoming an entrepreneur will not be simple; however, he outcome will be advantageous. Take a deep breath and enjoy the voyage. Through my experience, any Nurse inspired to open a business should first surround yourself around positive people who are genuinely there to cheer you along the way. My school would have closed two years ago if I didn't have cheerleaders uplifting me. Research the business in mind in depth and if possible, connect with other business owners that are established in that realm. The right people will be placed in the right places to help you along the journey. Trust in yourself and God. Hold on to your dream tight, it's yours. The most important tip is to pray and ask God to guide your footsteps, throughout your journey to success.

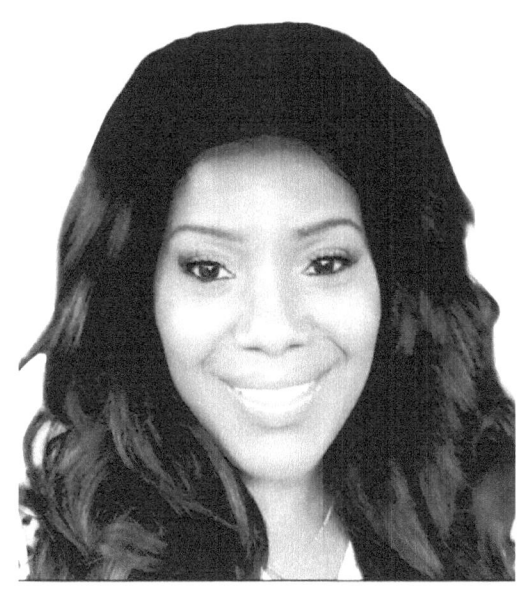

About the Author

Born in New Orleans, Louisiana, known as "The Big Easy", there was nothing that came easy to this southern raised beauty. Infatuated with fashion and style, her dream was to move to New York after high school and become a fashion designer and stylist, but growing up in the Lower Ninth Ward of New Orleans was challenging. As a teen, being subjected to observing friends dropping out of high school and becoming pregnant was all too common. Succumbing to her own pregnancy at the age of eighteen and becoming a mom to a little boy, Melanie McCrary- Fuller was determined to overcome the stereotypes and myths plagued amongst young women in her situation. With her dream of moving to New

York on the backburner, Melanie would work at retail stores and even venture into employment as a sheriff deputy. But one day a friend would ask her to accompany her to take a four-week Certified Nursing Assistant course that would take her on a career journey well worth it. Melanie would later become a Registered Nurse, BSN, after climbing the ladder as a Certified Nursing Assistant. Empowered by the many Nurses with whom she worked side by side, Melanie decided to further her medical career; not only did she become a Practical Nurse, but she would later receive two Nursing degrees. After working almost twenty years in healthcare and three kids later, Melanie was ready for change; so with her last child just a year old, she began to plan to open a Nursing training school. With lots of prayer, the help of her husband, and a 401k plan, the school was born. Melanie is not just a nurse building someone else's success; she is the owner of Advance Nursing Training, where she is building her success and legacy. When she's not managing the school, she's fulfilling the role of a Hospice Director of Nursing/Consultant. She also teaches the Train the Trainer course for Nurses interested in teaching Nursing Assistants. Dedicated to helping other Nurse Entrepreneurs, she provides individual consultations for Nurses interested in opening a proprietary school. When she's not indulging in Nursing and business, she is a wife, mom, and mentor.

To contact author:

Melaniemccraryant@gmail.com

IG: @advancenursingtraining

IG@the_nurse_connect

BEAUTY, BRAINS, AND BUSINESS

BY
Shawanna Guillory, FNP-BC

Chances are you're reading this book because you're a Nurse and you want to open your own business. If you're like me, you feel or have felt some guilt over wanting to leave the traditional Nursing roles. That's normal. But the truth is Nurses and entrepreneurship go perfect together. We possess all the skills necessary to be successful in business. We're smart, adaptable, good listeners, have excellent communication skills…. Shall I continue? And we possess valuable knowledge and experience that is in high demand. But if you've goggled anything related to opening a business, then you've encountered all the reasons not to. So, I applaud your determination to move forward despite the obvious risks. All of us have our individual reasons for wanting to pursue entrepreneurship, but I would be remiss if I didn't share with you a few tips that are important for everyone to know prior to heading out on that journey. The process isn't straight and narrow. Everyone's process is different. There's never a right time and you will encounter obstacles along the way. Expect it! I've found that researching the area of business that interests you as much as possible is important; and learning from others that have accomplished what you're attempting to do helps tremendously. So, here's MY story on becoming a business owner. I hope you find areas you can relate to, learn from, and implement on your journey.

Let me begin by acknowledging my excitement to be among the group of Nurse Practitioners that hold the #2 spot for best occupations in the United States. Yaaayyyy! Currently, I'm working as a Family Nurse Practitioner, performing in-home risk assessments for a major insurance carrier in addition to building my empire. But my career in Nursing began eighteen years ago as Certified Nursing Assistant. I wish I could say that being in the Nursing profession has been a childhood dream of mine. The truth is, I had no real plans or goals for my life past high school graduation. You see, I grew up in a family stricken with poverty and drug addiction. My mother worked various small jobs to keep us afloat. Although I admired her work ethic and determination, I had no real positive role models in my life. Dysfunction was normal in my household. So, there were no conversations regarding college, employment, or money. And it's not that I didn't have an idea of which path I would take; I had no thoughts about pursuing college or a career after graduation. Still today, my mom says she didn't think I would either; however, my senior year in high school proved to be a turning point in my life.

During my junior year, I recall seeing a group of seniors wearing colorful scrubs every day. They would leave school every morning and return mid-day to join their regular classes. I was curious to find out how I could do the same thing my senior year. After some investigation, I learned they were attending a nearby vocational school that offered a Nurse Aide training program. I signed up with the expectation of sailing through my senior year. To my surprise, I loved every aspect of caring for elderly patients. It was very rewarding and I felt like I made a difference in someone's life. In addition, my clinical instructor was the epitome of a great Nurse and Nurse educator. I had a fervent desire to emulate her. She became my first positive role model. It was in that Nurse Aide training program that I discovered the endless opportunities of the Nursing profession. Because of this life changing experience, I decided to further my education in Nursing and continue until I became a Nurse Practitioner.

I have always had an affinity to the elderly. Although I did not embrace it initially. There was and remains a stigma about Nurses not being considered "real Nurses" unless they worked on the medical/surgical floor before venturing out to other specialties. So, after I completed my LPN program, I applied at several hospitals for a position on the medical/surgical floor but to no avail. And I refused to apply at any Nursing home. After two months of being unemployed, I received a phone call regarding a part-time position at a local Nursing home. I accepted the job and the rest is history.

Moving forward, every position I've held was specific to the elderly population, which included skilled Nursing facilities, home health agencies, and medical house calls. Fast-forward eighteen years, I've gained extensive knowledge on the care and treatment of this population. I've witnessed firsthand the issues affecting their care. The issue that concerns me the most is the inadequate quality of care millions of elderly patients receive at home and in long-term care facilities. It was an issue when I initially entered the Nursing profession and remains a growing crisis. Those responsible for making a difference (good or bad) in the quality of care that patients receive is the staff that provides the care. You cannot address the quality of care given without addressing the staff that provides it. Certified Nursing Assistants (CNA's) provide up to 90% of that direct patient care. They are responsible for feeding, toileting, and bathing patients; but their role extends beyond those basic care services. Some of their additional responsibilities include performing lifesaving CPR/Heimlich maneuver, utilizing skin precautions (turning/repositioning) to prevent costly pressure ulcers and related complications, and documentation of vital information that impacts a patient's healthcare plan.

Due to their extensive contact with patients, CNA's are most likely the first healthcare team member to identify issues or changes with a patient. Consequently, they become the bridge between the patient and the Nurses/MD's. Their behavior and care directly impacts the patient's health. This is vital to the daily operations of any healthcare facility. Despite the significance of the CNA's role to healthcare, their value has diminished throughout the profession and society. In addition, they are plagued with issues which I believe negatively impact the quality of care provided to elderly patients. Studies have shown that increasing turnover rates, inadequate training, poor wages, understaffing, and higher risk for injuries result in poor outcomes for the elderly.

After witnessing the issues the elderly population and CNA's have faced over the years, it was evident that things needed to change. These issues have become the foundation of my businesses. It has become my mission to improve the quality of care provided to elderly patients. I believe that education, advocacy, and recognition will elevate the status and performance of our Certified Nursing Assistants. In return, a higher quality of care will be provided to the elderly population.

Another issue I've noticed among the elderly population is lack of transportation. More specifically, lack of transportation to medical appointments. It is a huge problem among the elderly population, especially the low-income patients. Most of them don't own a vehicle or multiple family members share one. Some patients are unable to drive and don't have any family/friends nearby to assist with transportation. This has been cited as a barrier to healthcare access. It leads to rescheduled or missed appointments, delayed care, and missed or delayed medication use. As a Nurse, I've witnessed some patients waiting until health issues worsen to get a ride to hospital by ambulance and this becomes their only access to healthcare. As a NP, I've provided medical house calls due to their inability to obtain transportation to and from a clinic. Without transportation, patients are unable to address changes in their health, which has proven fatal in some cases.

The problem is monumental and has serious health consequences that lead to poor management of chronic illnesses and poorer outcomes. We can provide the best care in the world, but it doesn't matter if the patient has no way to get to it. It is evident that this needs to change. Again, these issues have become the foundation for each business idea I pursue. So, I created Premier Transportation Services, LLC. I am in the process of hiring drivers and getting them approved by the state which is required for Medicaid reimbursement. My plan is to offer transportation, specifically for senior citizens, but also to anyone with a need to and from medical appointments. Research has shown that majority of the elderly population lose interest in living and battle depression once driving privileges are taken way; therefore, I plan to expand the business eventually to include non-medical transportation which would include grocery stores, hair salons, church, or family.

The idea of opening a business came after many years of contentment with working as a RN. Most of us are content, right? Until something happens that forces change. Don't get me wrong. The Nursing profession is very rewarding, but it does not come without its challenges. After years of dealing with long work hours, excess amounts of paperwork, holiday shifts, and spending time away from my family, I decided I needed to make a change. At that point, I knew I did not want to retire doing what I was doing. I wanted to be more present in my relationships. I wanted to create memories with my family. I didn't want anyone having control over when I can take a vacation, what days I could or couldn't work, and how much money I can make. Initially, I did not put forth any effort into bringing my plan to fruition. I was under the impression that it would take more money than I had to start any business which is one of the main reasons so many of us fail to move forward with opening a business. I also failed to do any research. I remember thinking that becoming a Nurse Practitioner would be my golden ticket to opening a business. I would have the skills and financial ability to open a clinic of my own and I would still be doing something I loved.

Surprisingly, after graduating as a Nurse practitioner, opening a clinic was the last thing I wanted to do. Although working in a clinic offered structured hours and holidays off, I decided I wanted more freedom and flexibility. Besides, my passion was caring for the elderly population and working in a clinic would not allow me to fulfill that need. This decision delayed my plan of becoming a business owner. I needed more time to ponder with other ideas that would enable me to utilize my degree while serving the elderly population.

Meanwhile, I landed the perfect job (or so I thought), making house call visits to elderly patients that were unable to leave the home to see a medical doctor/Nurse Practitioner for their primary care needs. I was expecting a salary of at least 90K with benefits. Instead, I was making about half of that without any benefits. Immediately, I knew this offer was not beneficial for me. I made more money as a Registered Nurse. Obtaining employment as a Nurse Practitioner is not an easy task; after all, it took five months to get hired by this employer. For this reason, I decided to cut my losses and gain some experience until I could find a better offer. After about a year of living paycheck to paycheck, a better offer did present itself. I was presented with the opportunity to work for a local company providing the same services. The position included an improved benefits package with a salary comparable to other Nurse Practitioners. The salary would go into effect six months after my hire date. It was contingent upon reimbursement from Medicare and private insurance. In the meantime, I agreed to the salary equivalent to a Nurse yet again. What was I thinking?

In my defense, I believed in the potential success of this company like it was my own. The services we provided were and remain in high demand. I wanted to assist the owner in rebuilding and expanding her company to provide services to as many elderly patients possible. In addition, I had faith that the result would be worth my initial sacrifices. Over the next six months, I worked tirelessly to rebuild her company through networking, direct marketing, and providing outstanding medical care. Just prior to the effective date of my agreed upon salary, financial issues began to arise between the owner and her investors. Unbeknownst to me, their financial issues could not be resolved and the company began to dissolve. I never received the salary I was promised. Two days prior to the official close of business, I was informed that the company was closing and my position would be terminated. I was devastated that this was the outcome after putting in so much time and making significant sacrifices financially and personally. I wasn't given enough time to seek alternative employment leaving my future uncertain as it related to my finances. This was my defining moment.

The last two years had been filled with lies, broken promises, and living paycheck to paycheck instead of the happiness and financial freedom I envisioned. I couldn't imagine the thought of living this way on a long-term basis. I refused to invest my time in any other businesses as much as I had unless it was my own. Eventually, I was hired with another company that could accommodate my financial needs; however, my personal life continued to suffer. My life was consumed with this job. I was on the road all day seeing patients and on the computer all evening doing documentation. I did have a conversation with my boss about making some changes. That was a waste of time. Have you ever noticed that when your employer needs you to make changes, we bend and get it done? But when the roles are reversed, the outcome is different. It makes me so angry.

They say if you don't build your own dream someone will hire you to build theirs. And that's exactly how I felt. I was being used to help build someone's dream who could care less about my struggles and issues. This inspired me even more to make the switch from employee to employer. By this time, I was desperate to create an action plan that I could implement to take me on the path I've envisioned. My passion for Nursing and the elderly led me to create an independent Nurse Aide training program. It was a no brainer, right? I often wondered how I hadn't thought of this idea sooner.

Obviously, I needed time to work on opening my own business. The solution was easy. I had to find another job that wouldn't require as much of my time. This job would also need to have equal or better pay to my previous job. It would help fund the startup process of my businesses. I didn't want to start off in debt by getting a business loan. Nothing is wrong with getting a business loan if that's what you need; it's just that owning a business is risky. I just felt more comfortable holding off on that with my first business. So, I prayed for this dream job. And God made it so. It seemed too good to be true. I questioned HR if this position was legit and it was. I left my full-time salaried position to work as an independent contractor.

The thought of leaving the security of a salaried position gave me anxiety as it does to most people. This is another circumstance holding people hostage from pursuing their dreams. I had to push past it. My desire to live the life I choose was stronger than my fear of failure and insecurities. I know many don't get this opportunity, but working as an independent contractor allowed me to have more time and complete control over my schedule and pay. It gave me an idea of what it would feel like to take that leap into entrepreneurship. I had faith it would all work out and it has. Finally, Premier Healthcare Training Solutions, LLC was created.

EDUCATION

As previously stated, I created my own Nurse Aide training program, but not just another Nurse Aide training program. My goal is to train and send CNA's out in the workforce who are compassionate, knowledgeable, and have a genuine desire to be in this profession. To achieve this goal, I extended my program over four weeks (instead of the two-week minimum), shortened the class periods to allow for increased retention of the information, and offered smaller classes to allow for increased attentiveness to each student's needs. I plan to offer the program in-house and on-site at long term care facilities. I have received approval of my program by the state of Louisiana. I'm planning to officially open for business in the fall with pending licensure as a proprietary school.

ADVOCACY

One of the things I've inherited as a Nurse Practitioner is a bigger platform. Also, the ability to speak to people whom I wouldn't have the opportunity to otherwise. I want to use my platform to bring about change. If the difficult decision is made to place a family member in long-term care, I want them to feel assured that they will be well taken care of. And that difficult decision could be ours any day. Long-term care facilities have a bad reputation as they relate to the care residents receive. Millions of dollars are being spent on preventable emergency room visits and hospital admissions. CNA's are key to the vitality of any healthcare facility, yet they have one of the lowest paid occupations. In Louisiana, there are no mandated Nurse Aide to resident ratios. I plan to use my voice to increase awareness and facilitate change in compensation and working conditions by speaking with my local public officials about these issues. It is my belief that making positive changes in these areas will have a direct positive impact on the care the elderly population receives.

RECOGNITION

Have your heard? People who feel appreciated always go the extra mile. National Nursing Assistants' Week 2017 is approaching. Do you as Nurses know the dates? It is June 15-22. Although it should be done on a regular basis, it's the perfect time for everyone to share their appreciation for Nursing Assistants and recognize the value they bring to the healthcare team. I want to see the community and more employers/staff recognizing the value and contributions Nursing Assistants bring to healthcare. I challenge every Nurse who reads this book to implement some form of recognition program or event at your facility. It is our patients who are suffering and it is our job to advocate for them.

To be a part of the change that is needed, I am giving an appreciation luncheon for some of the local CNA's in my community. To ensure that only the Nursing Assistants who truly deserve to be recognized attend the event, I selected different facilities and had the DON and/or CNA supervisor select the top three from their organization to attend and represent their facility. There will be speakers, awards, prize giveaways, and a catered lunch. In addition, I have some Nurse volunteers that will be serving the Nursing Assistants. Be on the lookout for pictures and videos from the event on my social media pages.

I would be remiss if I didn't put this out there. Social media will have you thinking it's so easy. Anyone can be a business owner. And you're not a "boss" unless you own a business. I don't agree with that. The sad truth is that owning a business is not for everyone. Some people will not and cannot handle the many sacrifices that come along with entrepreneurship. And successful people do exist who remain in corporate America. It is difficult and huge risks are involved. Did you know that half of small business startups fail within the first year? Such harsh statistics. And money isn't the only investment. Running a startup into profitability will require many hours of your time. Your relationships will suffer. You and only you become responsible for compensating employees regardless of the profitability of the business. And the stress of managing employees and being responsible for all decisions is enough to make you have a change of heart. But that's what makes us (entrepreneurs) different from the rest. We understand that although there are rewards of being your own boss and creating your own business, it is a difficult and complicated journey. And our passions allow us to persevere. Now if this didn't scare you off, chances are you have what it takes and you're ready for this entrepreneur life. So, this advice is for you.

There's no better time than now to start that business you've been dreaming about. Remember Rome wasn't built in a day. You may not be able to quit your job to work on your business and fund it today, but consistently taking small steps will lead to you accomplishing your business goals. Stay persistent. Many of us have our business ideas in mind already. For those who are undecided, there are many avenues and business opportunities unique to Nurses. The options are unlimited and we have an advantage over the general public due to our knowledge and experience. Some examples include education, consulting, and staffing. Most importantly though, think about issues you're most passionate about. What problems can you solve? Once you determine this, learn as much as you can about your niche. You should be an expert in your area of business. Then, educate yourself on the steps necessary to start your specific type of business. Don't be afraid to do what others aren't doing. Be strong enough to stand alone.

There will be times where you must do things you probably hate doing. For me, that would be public speaking. But no one can explain my purpose or pitch my business better than me. Initially, money may be tight but be willing to pay for the knowledge that will take you and your business to the next level. Don't expect anyone to invest in you if you aren't willing to invest in yourself. Just choose your investments wisely. One of these investments should be a coach, mentor, or accountability partner. Networking at social events and on social media makes it easier to find one that aligns with your goals. It helps tremendously to have support from someone who understands what you're going through. Entrepreneurship can get lonely at times. No one ever told me that. Sometimes I wish I had a business partner to share the responsibility and decision making with. It gets stressful doing it alone at times. I'm considering having someone to talk to or just vent helps me get through these tough times for my next business startup.

Professional networking is challenging but vital to the success of your business, particularly if you run or plan to run a small business. You will need connections to succeed in your business. Professional networking connects you with people and all their connections as well. This can lead to many new business opportunities, customers, and partnerships. Don't be fooled into thinking this cannot be done prior to opening your business. My CNA school isn't open yet, but I have already contacted and introduced myself and my business to most of the Administrators and Director of Nursing of the long-term care facilities in my community. My CNA appreciation luncheon will be the beginning of relationships with some of the top Nursing assistants in my community. Be proactive and have a plan. Finally, embrace any failures you experience and use them as opportunities to learn and grow from. Pick yourself up. Dust yourself off. And keep pushing! You can do this!

I have no doubt that at least one of our stories has ignited a fire in you to move forward with whatever your dreams are. No dream or goal is too big. Have you heard the saying "If your dreams don't scare you, they aren't big enough"? This is so true. It is all possible, but you must be willing to put in the work. We need to show the world that we are more than duck lips and selfies. Be pretty with a purpose. Let's set the example for our future Nurses on how we can be beautiful and have the brains to be CEO's of successful businesses as well.

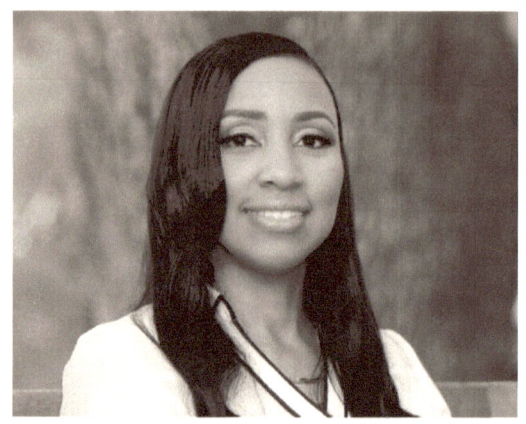

About the Author

Shawanna Guillory resides in Opelousas, Louisiana. Her career in nursing began at the age of eighteen working as a Nursing Assistant. While advancing her education, she gained valuable experience working in various settings for elderly patients including home health, skilled nursing units, and nursing homes. Ultimately, she obtained her Masters of Science Degree in Nursing from Southern University and A & M College. She is currently employed as an independent contractor with a major insurance carrier performing risk assessments. Over the past eighteen years, she has gained comprehensive knowledge in the care and treatment of elderly patients and the issues that affect their care. Her passion to improve the quality of care they receive inspired her to create Premier Healthcare Training

Solutions, LLC. It will offer training programs to become certified in CPR and as a nursing assistant. The expected grand opening is Fall 2016. Her goals are to assist in improving the quality of care elderly patients receive and changing the negative perception of nursing assistants in healthcare and society through education, advocacy, and recognition.

To Contact the Author:

Phone: 337-384-9219

Email: shawannag.fnp@gmail.com

Twitter: @TheNursepreneur

Instagram: @shawannag_thefnp

ALWAYS ON DUTY

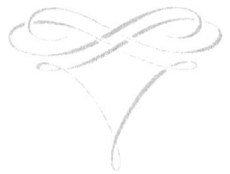

BY

Lakesha Reed-Curtis MSN, RN

So you are a Nurse and now you want more? I totally get it. I was once in your shoes, wanting more and just trying to figure out a way to live out my dreams. Six years later, I am doing just that. Let me give you a little information about myself before I dive in. I am Lakesha Reed-Curtis MSN, RN and the President/owner of Allied Health Academy, Medical Solutions Academy, Inc., which was founded in 2011. I also recently started Dream ChasHers, a women's empowerment group that encourages you to chase your dreams while having a tribe of women to back you. I have an amazing nine-year old son, KeShaun, and a beautiful baby girl, Madison, and have been married to my adoring husband Terrel for two years. I have been a Registered Nurse for fourteen years and received both my Bachelor and Master degrees in Nursing at Winston-Salem State University.

Now if you want to know why I chose to be a Nurse, let me tell you where I received my initial inspiration. I cannot remember my exact age, but I was around eleven or twelve when the idea was brought to me. My cousin Courtney and I were at my grandmother's house and he had a nosebleed, so I ran to his aid. I remember my grandmother saying, "Girl, you should be a Nurse." That's right, you know how grandmothers are; any little thing you do right, she cheers you on. She spoke that destiny over my life for the rest of my teenage years; so, when it was time for me to go to college, my major was Nursing. Thank God I loved it. It's funny how things happen in your life and how you can speak things into existence. Ironically, I don't remember my cousin ever having another nosebleed. Call me crazy, but maybe God allowed that nosebleed to happen at that particular time so that my grandmother could speak over me. Honestly, if I didn't have that programmed in my head for so many years, I don't know where I would be or what I would be doing. Thanks grandma!!!

When it was time for college, I left home for Old Dominion University and managed to stay for one whole semester. Yep...only one semester. I was extremely homesick and knew the environment wasn't one I wanted to adjust to. I came home for Christmas break and never went back, except to retrieve my things. So here I was back at home with my family looking at me crazy, wondering what I was going to do next. I applied at my local community college and was accepted into the Practical Nursing Program. I couldn't afford to go straight into RN school because of the time frame it required. I needed to be finished with school quickly so I could start working in the field. Once accepted, my grandma was very ecstatic. I remember telling her that one day I may open my own school. It was a joke at the time, but look at me now! That is a prime example of putting your dreams out into the universe and seeing them come to fruition. I truly believe that with all my heart. Before you go any further, speak it out in the atmosphere your heart's desires and watch God work. Keep Him close. That's the first step.

When I completed the Practical Nursing Program, I gained employment at a local nursing home. I was allowed to work 90 days until I sat for my exam. I was so happy, I was making money and living large and in charge. I went to take my exam and I failed, not once but three times. It was one of the most devastating things in my life. Each time I failed I vowed that I would not retake the test. As soon as those ninety days rolled around for me to test again, I was there hoping to pass. During this time I was taking prerequisite courses to gain admission into a RN program. I had and still have a huge amount of faith. Finally passing on the fourth try I decided to move to Hampton, Virginia for a change of scenery several months later. I decided to purse my RN degree while I was there. So three years later I received my Associates degree from a local community college. Upon the completion of my studies, I returned back to Danville, VA. I then received my Bachelors from Winston Salem State University. After completing my studies for my Bachelor in Nursing, I eventually moved to Charlotte, North Carolina in hopes of creating more opportunities for my son and I. With this move came a new job opportunity as Assistant Director of Nursing for a company in the Concord area. I was making a pretty decent salary with this company, but I just constantly felt like something was missing. I needed the freedom to live on the edge a little, take business risks, and make my own choices without the constraints of a set schedule or someone else's rules. I don't think people realize how working for someone else consumes your whole life; all areas are dictated by work because of that tight schedule that comes with it. I was sick of asking for paid time off to take vacations, have a "me" day, or even run errands! And let's be honest, thirty minutes is just not enough time to enjoy a nice lunch. I knew I couldn't work a regular nine to five job long-term and I needed to make a change quick!

Starting my own business had always been something I wanted to do, but I was skeptical of my own abilities and the great unknown of self-employment. It was time for me to stop feeling like I was missing the mark and do something about the unsettling feeling that had been haunting me daily. I just had to figure out what my niche was. I knew I wanted to help my community in a different way than what was already being provided. My main objective was to constantly learn and advance in whatever I chose to do with the goal of success as the common denominator. Most importantly, I wanted to be home with my son as much as possible once he started school.

I remember working the job as Assistant Director of Nursing, making a pretty decent salary, but all the while realizing this was not enough sustainable income to take care of my son and me. I mean life was good, don't get me wrong; but I knew it could be better. I needed it to be better. During the years that I worked from nine to five, I found myself deeply craving the ability to spend more time with my child. By the time I picked him up from daycare, it would be dark outside and the day was already over. It was during those times I set a goal to be at home with him daily before he started Kindergarten; at the time, he was only two so I had a little leeway before he started school. I would sit around and just pray for a business idea to come to me, all the while never losing focus or hope in my dreams.

One night as I was lying in bed with KeShaun, the idea of selling scrubs came to me. In that moment, I hugged him so tight and began to jump up and down in the bed! I remember it all so well. I thought big, but started small. I knew my dreams would not allow me to remain small and growth was in my future. I begin doing trade shows at local nursing homes and sold scrubs to most of my co-workers and Nursing friends. Little did I know, this was the start of my entrepreneurial journey! My best friend's mother, Sandra Estes, allowed me to have my first trade show at her Nursing facility. My good girlfriend would travel with me in my Camry to facilities that were two hours away, all squished up and surrounded by the scrubs I was carrying up the road to sell. We still laugh about it to this day! I can look back and laugh at it now, but back then this had become my livelihood and my ticket to working for myself. At the time, I was still working my fulltime job. So future nurse entrepreneurs, it's always good to have a side hustle. Shoot, I still will go to a local nursing facility and sell a scrub or two out of my trunk. Never get to comfortable that you lose your hustle. It just goes to show, it doesn't matter how small you start as long as you start somewhere.

I always liked education and knew I would one day go in this direction in my career; however, I never actually imagined I would be the owner of a school.]As a graduate of Nursing school, I quickly recognized that Nursing programs were becoming a trend in North Carolina. This piqued my interest since I had always had the desire to teach. I quickly began researching the requirements and qualifications necessary to become a Nursing instructor. This turned into me submitting my application not only to teach but also to open my own school! Ironically, I was terminated from my job as Assistant Director of Nursing in November 2010 and Medical Solutions Academy opened in April 2011. Who would have known that I could get the ball rolling with just a five-month time frame? God is amazing! To this day I wonder if I would not have gotten fired, would I have been brave enough to quit the job and follow my dream? It's hard for me to say; but at the time my back was against the wall, so I did what I needed to do. I refused to let another individual or company determine the fate of my family and me. In my eyes, I had no other options so I stepped out on faith and started MSA.

When I was terminated from my job, I was already in the process of submitting my paperwork to the Board of Nursing to have my Nurse Aide program approved. During this time my life was very stressful. I was in the process of buying a home, I had just lost my job, and my lease was running out on my apartment. The broker of my home was telling me to find another job so I would not lose my house, but I refused. I had faith and was determined God would see me through; however, I did find a part-time job teaching at a local Nurse Aide school. I only worked there for about two months because my program was quickly approved. Not to mention, I had received the credentials I needed to move into my new home and had started that process as well.

To move forward with my program, I had to have a building to hold the courses. For some, an obstacle like this would steer them off course; but once again I kept the faith and allowed God to steer me in the right direction. A local realtor allowed me to use the address on my paperwork until I was approved without paying anything. See how God works things out when you choose not to stress and let him lead the way? So as soon as my program was approved with a pending site visit, I literally had one week to set up my school completely. I had been purchasing equipment along the way, so the process was not too strenuous. Now my first building/school was very small. It consisted of three rooms, which were not connected. I painted those rooms my favorite royal blue color and was on my way. I was so proud. I was also thankful to God most of all for seeing this through. My major goal was to be at home with my son daily once he started Kindergarten; but I had the opportunity be home once he started Pre-K, which was even sooner than planned. God is amazing!

Once my school opened in Danville, Virginia, I was blessed with a full class from the start. I truly believe this was because I put a little buzz in the community a couple of months before I opened. You know how some people say don't tell others your dreams? Well, I am the opposite. If you know your dreams are going to happen, then tell someone. You don't want to open a business and not have the word out to the public that you are about to open. Word of mouth is always a good marketing tool especially in a tight knit community. Just remember, any time you tell people your dreams, there will always be a few who will try to deter you from following your desired journey; but never let anyone else determine your path in life. You can do whatever you set your mind out to do!

When I initially opened MSA, I had a secretary and worked sixteen hours a day for the first year. I taught the day and evening classes. I was so tired, but it was the most fulfilling thing I had ever done. For once, I really was the BOSS. Now I don't want you to think that being a Nursepreneur is all glitz and glamour. It is hard work, but dreams do become a reality if you put in the effort. Despite the time and effort I was putting into teaching these classes, the reward for my work was priceless. I don't want you to get confused and think those times will not come when you have no one to talk to and you are in the closet crying. You know what I mean, the ugly cry. Trust me you will be broke at times either because business is simply slow or you have just invested a lot of money in your business; but let me tell you this, money should be the least of your worries. You have the money in your brain and you will reap the benefits of your labor sooner than you think. Just get started. Slow progress is better than no progress. You don't want to have any what-ifs lingering in your head.

After the first year of business, I was finally able to hire staff and return to my home in North Carolina. Yep, I opened a business two hours away from my home in Charlotte back in my hometown. Now this part of my entrepreneur journey is still the hardest to manage. If my staff gets low, I may have to stay away from home for a couple of days. If things go array, I cannot be there in the blink of an eye because I live too far away. I sometimes think about moving closer to my establishment, but that would defeat the purpose of being an entrepreneur. I like the freedom entrepreneurship establishes; therefore, I feel as though I should be able to work from anywhere in the world.

Medical Solutions Academy now has a Nurse Aide, Medication Aide, Pharmacy Technician, Medical Office Assistant, Medical Assistant, a CPR course, and a Phlebotomy Technician program. I am currently in the process of obtaining a Practical Nursing Program. Boy oh boy, that process has been long and arduous; I could write an entire book on that task alone. Let's just say some things don't come to you as fast or as smooth as you want them too; but when you keep the faith, they will come to pass. Never give up!!!

Although being an entrepreneur has granted me the desired freedom to work as I please, we all know being the boss is not easy! Couple that with being a mom and a wife and you have reached a completely new level of being on demand for your time. Every woman will have her own set of rules and guidelines she lives by to balance her everyday life. My one and only rule is God first, then family, and THEN business. I live by this and try my best to follow this day in and day out. Anytime I tend to stray from this line of order, it seems like my whole world turns upside down. When things tend to go wrong, I check myself to make sure I'm following my golden rule. If I find that I've switched that order, I'll immediately start praying and ask God to align my vision to his again. My purpose in starting my business was given to me through the talents with which God blessed me and He will forever come first in my life. My family is and will always be my main priority on Earth; therefore, although my business is my baby, it will always come third in my life.

Giving up honestly has never been a thought to cross my mind. I do have those moments when I say forget this, I am going to find a job; however, I get over that in 20-30 minutes flat. Who would I be kidding? I am an entrepreneur by nature and at heart. The process does get hard and you will face a lot of adversity. Sometimes it comes from those closest to you. I have moments when I question myself. Who am I to start a school and have all of these big dreams and goals? But as I knock those goals out, I am quickly reminded of who I am… Lakesha Reed-Curtis, a dreamer and a doer. I honestly believe there is nothing I cannot accomplish with God, the right team, and the right mindset. This is something you must remember - nothing great can be done alone and you have to pay to play. Don't try to get everything done for free. Words that my husband always tells me are, "You get what you pay for." This is so true. Invest, Invest, Invest in your business! I cannot stress this enough. It is also important to have a good lawyer and accountant in your corner early in business. I wish someone would have told me that before getting started, but this is one of the many lessons I have learned along the way.

I also suggest having multiple streams of income. Medical Solutions Academy is my bread and butter; however, I like to invest in real estate on the side. Renovating properties has become a passion of mine and has allowed extra money to flow into my life so I can have more room to grow Medical Solutions Academy. It is a lot of work, but I love to see a place once deemed unsuitable for living transform into a warm and cozy place for someone to call their home. Just as with MSA, because I enjoy dabbling in real estate and renovating properties, it feels like less of a job and more of a destiny that God purposefully placed on my path.

You will face many obstacles on your journey to entrepreneurship, but passion will take you where you need to go. When you stay focused and put your all into your dreams, it begins to feel as if your back is against the wall. You will either fold and go back to working for someone else, or you will be driven that much more to continue on your pursuit of reaching your goals. No matter how difficult my journey may have gotten, turning back was never an option for me. I had my family depending on me and I was determined to not only be a good mom, but to also be present as much as possible. I already had the passion for Nursing; coupled with the desire to be at home with my kids as much as possible, these two factors gave me the motivation I needed to see my dreams come to fruition.

If you can control the way your mind thinks of being a Nursepreneur, I strongly believe you will make it through the process. Too often we allow self-doubt and fear creep into our minds and gain control of our thoughts. All of a sudden, what once seemed easy now seems impossible all because of negative thinking. We are our own biggest enemy in life. Next thing you know, you're convincing yourself not to quit your job and go into business for yourself because it seems illogical. If you focus on what could go wrong instead of all the things that are going right, then everything will fall apart quicker than you could ever imagine. You have to have faith in yourself and on the days you can't put faith in yourself, put it in God because there is absolutely nothing he cannot do. What is meant for you is for you and no one can deter you from receiving your blessings. I am constantly looking for new ways to build my empire and leave a legacy for my family therefore, I'M ALWAYS ON DUTY to ensure I do just that.

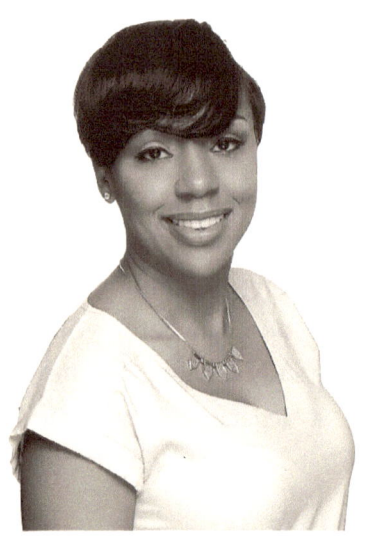

About the Author

Mrs. Lakesha Reed- Curtis, wife and mother of two, is a woman of action who Dreams Big and just decided to Chase Hers! She was born and raised in Danville, Virginia, but now currently resides in Charlotte, North Carolina with her loving family. Her focus in life has always been to find different avenues with the opportunity to provide services to the community. Her goal then became to provide higher education opportunities for students interested in the healthcare field to advance career wise in the future. By introducing Medical Solutions Academy to her community, she has become dedicated to empowering her community through educational programs that serve to make prospective health care workers prepared for employment in the medical field.

Lakesha Curtis has fourteen years of hands-on nursing experience and received both her Bachelor and Master degree from Winston-Salem State University. By establishing Medical Solutions Academy, she has gained adequate experience in the full process of operating and administrating successful medical certification programs from start to finish. She has had the opportunity to witness students complete these certification programs over the course of the last six years. Her educational program has expanded over the years and now includes Nurse Aide, Phlebotomy Technician, Pharmacy Technician, Medical Assistant, Medication Aide, Medical Office Assistant, CPR Certification, and soon LPN. She has built this school from the ground up and enjoys playing such an important role in others' lives.

Constantly facing the demands of maintaining a family and a career simultaneously, Lakesha understood how difficult it is for some women to chase their own dreams. She saw the need to form a group of empowering women to keep each other motivated, which sparked the beginning of Dream ChasHers. She now hosts networking events and even held a vision board party to kick of the new year. She plans to host even more events in the future and build Dream ChasHers into another one of her empires. Although she may wear many titles, she wears them all effectively and efficiently while encouraging other women that they have the power to do the same.

To Contact The Author:

Dreamchashers.com

info@dreamchashers.com

Instagram @lakesha_curtis , @dream_chashers, @medicalsolutionsacademy

Facebook: Facebook.com/lakeshareed-curtis

THE JOURNEY: NURSING AND BEYOND

BY
Tiffany Jackson, LPN

As far back as I can remember I have always loved the medical field. As a child, I can remember enjoying the smells of my doctor's office during my visits. When I was younger, I had episodes where I would faint from low blood sugar. I remembered how nice and caring the Nurses were to me. The Nurses were attentive to me during my time of need and this is something that I have always remembered. Since I always knew that I wanted to be in the medical field, knowing which career path direction was a little more difficult. I thought about becoming a physician, physician assistant or respiratory therapist. It took many years and different experiences to decide on nursing as a career choice.

Prior to my medical career, I had various customer service based jobs, from working in a coffee shop to working as a customer service representative for a credit card company. I have always enjoyed helping other people, but I never felt that sense of fulfillment while working at these jobs. While I was going through this transitional period, my grandmother was diagnosed with breast cancer. I took her to her chemotherapy and radiation appointments. During this time, I could see first-hand how kind and knowledgeable the Nurses were and readily available when my grandmother had questions. The Nurses went out of their way to show and give support to my grandmother during this difficult period in time. This was when I decided on nursing as a career choice.

I saw an advertisement in the local newspaper about an upcoming certified nursing assistant (CNA) course. After completing the CNA program, I wanted to advance to another level. I completed the patient care technician course at Savannah Technical College. With the Patient Care Technician (PCT) program course, I was educated on the techniques of drawing blood, basic wound care, colostomy care, Foley catheter insertion and care and ecgs, just to name a few skills. After being taught these skills, I could work at the local hospital. My first job was on the Neurology/Neuro Step-Down unit. On this unit, we received individuals who had head or spinal cord injuries. It was important to understand proper body mechanics on how to turn patients during bed baths or for repositioning and the importance of knowing that not using those techniques can cause further injuries to the patient. I can remember taking care of my first patient with a halo apparatus after he broke his neck while diving in a pool. I was very nervous that I would cause more damage to his neck when I turned him. He was in a lot of pain from the screws and pins to his head. I relied on my PCT training regarding the proper body mechanics for turning and repositioning for this patient. Another situation that I remember, was a patient who had a head injury and who was confused and combative to the nursing staff. We would have to redirect this patient multiple times, which taught me patience and the importance of having it. Patience can be the key factor in determining if you will have a "good" or "bad" shift.

Many times, as an PCT I felt as if my job was not as important because the Nurse gave the medications that the doctors ordered to help the patients and most of what I did was take vitals and blood sugars, bathed patients, etc. I initially did not fully understand that my job was also important. Many times, I could see the patients before the Nurse and I could detect a change in the patient and alert the Nurse of the change. There was an older patient who had a low blood pressure, low oxygen levels in the 80s and her lips were blue. I immediately got the Nurse who could assess the patient and call the Rapid Response Team and she was taken down to the Intensive Care Unit (ICU). After that experience, I felt that I played a small role in helping to save that lady's life before a code blue situation occurred. This was when I fully understood the term of being the eyes and ears for the Nurses. Therefore, I have always appreciated the CNAs and PCTs because of experiences like these. As a PCT, I could spend more one on one time with the patient which gave me a little more insight on patient's home life or previous illnesses. I could find out that some of my patients were struggling between paying for their medications and buying food. I would notify the Nurse or social worker to get that patient some assistance to help them during the difficult period.

After working on the Neurology unit for a while, I could transfer to the emergency department, which was a Level One Trauma Center. I learned a lot and I loved going to work. Each day was always something new and different to learn. My favorite section to work in was Trauma and Cardiac. I believed that I enjoyed Trauma and Cardiac because I could learn so much from not only the Nurses but also the doctors and patients. Since the emergency department was a Level One Trauma Center, we received all the critical patients in the surrounding area. The range of patients that we received were from car accident victims, gun shot victims, strokes, and other critical patients from other hospitals. As a PCT at a Level One

Trauma Center, I was like a "sponge" trying to soak up all the knowledge that I possibly could. In the emergency department, I would sometimes work with a Nurse who was also a flight Nurse. She enjoyed teaching just as much as I did learning. She taught me about the signs and symptoms of many disease processes and the importance of labs and how the lab results would give a detail description of the patient's disease process. Many of the doctors also enjoyed teaching and quizzing you on disease processes. Being in this very rich learning environment further increased my desire to go into nursing, until I had an experience that made me rethink if I truly wanted nursing as a career choice.

There was an incident where a toddler was killed after being backed over by a vehicle. We worked on that toddler it seemed like forever until the toddler eventually died. Myself and another PCT had to help with making the toddler look "presentable" for the parents to see. We had to put 4x4 gauze and gauze bandages around the toddler's head where the brain was exposed. We had to remove the bloody sheet underneath and put a clean sheet under the toddler. I held the child while the other tech replaced the sheet. I stared at the toddler with disbelief that I was holding a dead child in my arms. I thought about how would I feel if that were my son. There were a lot of family and friend in the privacy room area in the back of the department. The doctor came in and introduced himself to the group. The family hung on every word as the doctor explained that every possible medical intervention was used to help the child. As the doctor began to apologize, I saw the mother fall on the floor and began to scream and sob. The mother's scream pierced my soul. It was extremely difficult to look at this and no amount of "I'm sorry for your loss" would be able to comfort those parents. When I went home that evening, I hugged my son even more tightly than I have before and I had difficulty sleeping that night. This incident made me questioned nursing as a career choice. I thought, "How can I comfort someone during such a difficult time in their life?" When I returned to work, I spoke with a Nurse who has been a Nurse for many years. She told me that she finds peace in knowing that she was providing comfort and care for someone during their time of need or their last moments in life. This gave me a new perspective towards helping individuals during their time of need. I began to think the same way and that was how I could get past that traumatic event of the child dying.

During the early 2000s, I began to dabble a little with having an online business. I would sell items on my website and also through one of the well-known auction sites. Even though I enjoyed having an online business it was a very stressful period of time for me. I eventually decided to close my online store. Also, during this time I began to feel the desire to advance my career to another level. I applied to Altamaha Technical College Licensed Practical Nurse program (now Coastal Pines Technical College). I did not think that I would get into the program even though I hoped and prayed I would. I was so nervous because it was a panel interview of four people. I was asked a range of questions from why I want to become a Nurse to how would I react in different situations. I was accepted into the program. I continued to work full-time by working 12-hour shifts on Friday through Sunday and I attended school Monday through Thursday while raising my young son at the time. I was so grateful for my family support during that time. After completing the Licensed Practical Nurse program, I moved to Virginia. My first job was a Charge Nurse position at a long-term care facility. This is where I met one of my best friends Bridgette; she was one of the most knowledgeable Nurses that I have ever known. From that position, I worked on a specialty care ventilator/tracheostomy unit where I met another best friend Kimberly, who is also a very knowledgeable Nurse.

After working there for about a year, I was able to get a Federal position at a local hospital working on the Oncology/Medical-Surgical unit. Working on this unit humbled me more than any other experience. When a person's life is coming to an end, many of the problems that people worry about will not be as important. When individuals are dying no one says "I wished I worked that overtime" or "I wish I paid those bills", people always say "I wish I spent more time with my family". Since I worked as an inpatient Nurse many of my patients were very sick due to infections and low blood count levels. On our unit when patients would die, they usually died in groups of three or four. This was very difficult to handle because I became very close to my patients and their family. I had episodes where I had to deal with the depressed feeling that I felt after their death. On my off days, I would think about my patients and wonder how well they are handling their treatments. When our patients would complete their treatment successfully it was like a huge celebration. Patients would invite their family members and friends to attend the event. Before the patient would leave the unit, there was a plaque that had wording celebrating the successful completion of the patient's oncology treatments. The patient would read the plaque out loud and then ring the bell three times. I loved seeing when a patient completed their treatments. This was always an exciting time for everyone on the unit. It gave the

Nurses a sense of accomplishment that they had helped someone during their time of need; and for the other patients seeing this celebration, it helped to increase their faith and determination to complete their treatments.

While working on this unit I experienced the government shutdown, because the nursing staff is considered essential personnel we were required to work without pay and prior to the shutdown, myself and many other staff members experienced being furloughed. Furlough is a decrease in working hours, instead of working 80 hours every two weeks I only worked 60 every two weeks. I did not have a second job or my online business to supplement my income. I was able to find a second job once the government reopened. It always remained in the back of my mind how I need to have another stream of income coming into my home. It was not until later that I was introduced to subscription box service.

The idea of my business started because one day after coming home from work I removed my socks and I saw where I needed a pedicure. I was so busy taking care of other people that I was not taking care of myself. I began to think, "If I, who loves pedicures, can put myself last, there must be other Nurses or medical professionals who are doing the same. I decided to develop The CareZONE Box, which is a monthly subscription box service for medical professionals. This box helps to promote relaxation and pampering for the medical professional. I believe that anyone can make a side hustle or passion into a business, it only takes effort and thoughtfulness to succeed. Another reason why I wanted another online business was for possibility of financial freedom of knowing that you can have money coming in without having to clock into a job.

When I decided on pursuing the subscription box service as a small business, I shopped around trying to determine which company I was going to use for my business. After narrowing down that company, trying to decide a name was difficult. My son and I came up names like the Medicine box, Med box to Treatment box. We finally narrowed it to The CareZONE Box. As medical professionals, the foundational basis of any medical career is care. When I send out my boxes to my customers I want them to know how much thoughtfulness and care was put into each box. I enjoy researching new products to introduce to my customers. I have a few small business companies that I network with to introduce their products to my customers. I enjoy working with these companies as it has taught me many valuable lessons with how to conduct business and contracts with other companies. I experience difficulty while designing my website. I had to learn about website coding, which was very difficult. It took a few months to finish my website; however, I was truly elated once it was complete.

A few key advises for anyone who wants to start a business is to first have passion and determination that your business will be successful. The individual must think positive in hopes that their business will be meaningful to other people. I have and will always believe that my business will be successful and meaningful if I keep God first and second the desire to offer great products to my customers at an affordable price. Another key advice is to be bold and step out into places that may make you feel uncomfortable. For example, if you believe a certain company or individual can help your business, be bold enough to ask them for their advices or other services that can help your business. If you don't try the answer will always be

No! When I first started my business, I had to reach out to other businesses that I believed would assist me with success within my business. I was extremely nervous because I was thinking that the company would not take me serious because I was just starting out. I had a few companies who did not respond back to me and I had many companies who did respond to my emails. Experiencing situations like this has increased my confidence to approach people and companies. I enjoy working with other small business owners as we try to work together to make each other's business successful. Also, usually if I buy bulk with a small business the amount that is considered bulk is smaller than working with a larger company's definition of buying bulk. Learning this valuable lesson early on assisted me with staying within budget and assisted with being able to provide various products at an affordable cost to my customers.

Another key is to ask a lot of questions. If there is something that you are unsure of, ask questions or Google it. I learned this lesson the hard way when the company that I ordered my boxes from took three weeks to process the order. This time did not include the time for shipping. I assume that it would have taken only a week to two weeks before shipping. Therefore, my very first box shipment was late. I had to pay extra money to have my boxes shipped overnight to me. I sent out emails to notify customers of this delay. This was a very embarrassing situation for me. Therefore it is very important to ask questions and not assume based on past experiences. The last and probably the most important key advice would be to stay organized. Always keep a notebook handy or enter information or questions into your phone that may arise throughout the day. I like to make notes on items that I need to follow up on or articles that I would like to read later. Anytime you have a business to manage there are so many things that you are responsible for; for example, increase in emails (personal and business) or many individuals contacting you for business opportunities to advance your business or to help promote their business. This shows how staying organized is very important for your business and daily life in general. As a business owner, you will need to keep a tight budget for accounting and tax purposes. Knowing what is coming in and going out within your business will help to keep your business running at an optimal level.

During my life, the many experiences and opportunities have made me into the person who I am today. Through the many hardship and trails that I have experienced in life has made me stronger person and Nurse in general. As I propel to my next level of nursing towards a Registered Nurse degree. I will take all my experiences from CNA up to LPN to assist with making myself more of a wiser and stronger Nurse. I will remain empathetic to situations and not just sympathetic, which will improve my outlook on life in general. Viewing situation from another person point of view will help you to see situations much clear. I will also use these experiences to make my business excel to another level. As I continue, working with other small businesses to make each other's business successful.

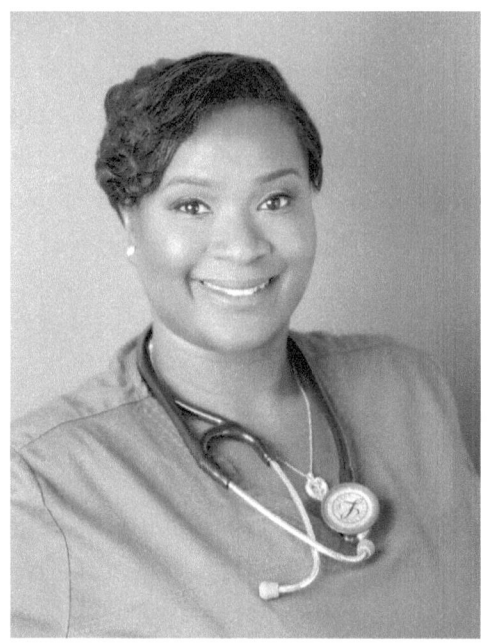

About the Author

Tiffany L. Jackson is a Licensed Practical Nurse who completed her degree at Altamaha Technical College (now called Coastal Pines Technical College). She is wound care certified and is currently working to be certified in many other areas of nursing. She is a member of the National Association for Practical Nurse Education and Services (NAPNES). Tiffany currently attends Savannah State University in Savannah, Georgia and Indiana State University in Terre Haute, Indiana with the hopes to complete the LPN to RN-BSN program. She has had various nursing jobs that ranged from Long Term Care to Medical/Surgical nursing. She is a current employee at the Ralph H. Johnson Veterans Affairs Medical Center at the clinic location in Savannah, Georgia. She is the owner and creator of The CareZONE Box, which is a monthly subscription service box for medical professional. This subscription box helps to promote relaxation and pampering. She has a son and her hobbies include traveling and reading.

To Contact The Author:

www.thecarezonebox.com

IG:@thecarezonebox

References

Benveniste, ALEXIS*Approximately 58,000 college students are homeless* https://www.aol.com/article/2015/07/24/approximately-58-000-college-students-are-homeless /21213755/

Boundless. "*The Biopsychosocial Model of Health and Illness.*" Psychology Boundless, 20 Sep. 2016. Retrieved 22 Apr. 2017 from https://www.boundless.com/psychology/textbooks/boundless-psychology-textbook/stress-and-health-psychology-17/introduction-to-health-psychology-85/the-biopsychosocial-model-of-healt

Bureau of Labor Statistics, U.S. Department of Labor. *Occupational Outlook Handbook*. 2011.http://www.bls.gov/ooh/healthcare/registered-nurses.htm.

Cimiotti, J., et al. (2012). Nurse staffing, burnout, and health care-associated infections. *American Journal of Infection Control, 40(6)*, 486-490

Missouri Department of Health and Senior Services, *Certified Medication Technician (CMT) Program*   http://health.mo.gov/safety/cnaregistry/cmt.php

The National Council of State Boards of Nursing, Inc. (NCSBN), *Application & Registration* https://www.ncsbn.org/index.htm

The National Law Center on Homelessness & Poverty *Homelessness in America: Overview of Data and
Causes*   www.nlchp.org/documents/Homeless_Stats_Fact_Sheet

Standard & Poor's Ratings Services, "*The U.S. Health Care Sector Outlook Is Demonstrating Resilience As 2016 Unfolds*." https://www.spratings.com/.../US_PF.../8ff75189-b5e0-41dc-b8ef-930f32d08f89

Statistic Brain, "*Homeless Poverty Statistics Data Number of homeless people in the US.*" Published: Mar 31, 2017 http://www.statisticbrain.com/homelessness-stats/

www.ingramcontent.com/pod-product-compliance
Lightning Source LLC
Chambersburg PA
CBHW031049180526
45163CB00002BA/751